TOTAL FITNESS AND NUTRITION AFTER 40: 2-IN-1 VALUE BUNDLE

THE 2 LIFE CHANGING BOOKS YOU NEED FOR STRENGTH, HEALTHY EATING HABITS AND MOTIVATION IN YOUR 40S, 50S, 60S AND BEYOND

NICK SWETTENHAM

WWW.NICKSWETTENHAMFITNESS.COM

© **Copyright Nick Swettenham 2022- all rights reserved**

The content contained within this book may not be reproduced, duplicated or transmitted without direct written permission from the author or the publisher.

Under no circumstances with any blame or legal responsibility be held against the publisher, or author, for any damages, reparation, or monetary loss due to the information contained within this book. Either directly or indirectly. You are responsible for your own choices, actions and results.

Legal Notice:

This book is copyright protected. This book is only for personal use. You cannot amend, distribute, sell, use, quote, or paraphrase any part, or the content within this book, without the consent of the author or publisher.

Disclaimer notice:

Please note, the information contained within this document is for educational and entertainment purposes only. All effort has been executed to present accurate, up to date and reliable, complete information. No warranties of any kind are declared or implied. Readers acknowledge that the author is not engaging in the rendering of legal, financial, medical or professional advice. The content of this book has been derived from various sources. Please consult a licensed professional before attempting any techniques outlined in this book.

By reading this document, the reader agrees that under no circumstances is the author responsible for any losses, direct or indirect, which are incurred as a result of the use of the information contained within this document, including, but not limited to, - errors, omissions or inaccuracies. The author is in no way responsible for any injuries that might occur as a result of using the exercises recommended in this book.

CONTENTS

TOTAL FITNESS AFTER 40

Introduction	13

1. AS WE AGE, WE CHANGE — 19
What's Happening to My Body?	19
What Fitness Can Do For You	28
The 7 Foundations of Total Fitness	30
Key Points	38

2. DEVELOPING A MINDSET FOR SUCCESS — 40
The Power of Visualization	42
SMART Goal Setting	43
Learning to Love Exercise	47
Building the Exercise Habit	49
Energy Systems	57
The Importance of Your Training Heart Rate	59
Key Points	62

3. STRENGTH - YOU ARE STRONGER THAN YOU KNOW! — 64
The Strength Training Pyramid	73
Movement Quality	74
Next up in the pyramid is Exercise Selection.	76
Exercise Selection	76
Intensity, Volume, Frequency	80
Progression	82
Rest Intervals / Tempo	83
Specifics/ Details	86
Strength Training in Practice	86
Sample Workouts.	90

Warming Up / Cooling Down ... 90
Summary ... 93

4. FLEXIBILITY - STRETCH TO IMPRESS ... 95
What is Flexibility? ... 96
Flexibility Benefits ... 96
Why We Become Less Flexible With Age ... 97
Most Common Flexibility Issues for the Elderly ... 98
Gender Differences ... 99
Types of Stretching ... 100
Flexibility Testing ... 102
Stretching Recommendations ... 105
16 Great Static Stretches ... 105
Yoga for Flexibility ... 110
Summary ... 112

5. MOBILITY - MOVE IT OR LOSE IT! ... 114
The Importance of Mobility ... 114
Typical Mobility Issues ... 117
Improving Your Mobility ... 118
Self Myofascial Release ... 119
Dynamic Stretching ... 123
Mobility Drills ... 125
Summary ... 130

6. STABILITY - FINDING THE BALANCE ... 131
The Stability-Mobility Continuum ... 132
Keeping our Body Stable ... 134
Improving your Stability ... 136
Lower Body ... 137
Upper body ... 140
Adding Stability into Gym Routines ... 142
Summary ... 146

7. AGILITY - NOW THE FUN BEGINS! ... 147
Agility ... 147
Agility Training Benefits ... 149

Agility Training Applied: Plyometrics   151
Summary   156

8. ENDURANCE - DON'T STOP ME NOW!   157
Never Give Up!   157
What is Endurance?   158
Reversing the Endurance Trend   160
Warm up   163
Dynamic Stretching Routine   165
Shoulder Circles   166
Cooldown   167
Improving Muscular Endurance   170
Summary   171

9. NUTRITION: YOU ARE WHAT YOU (CHOOSE) TO EAT   173
Nutrition and Aging   174
Macro & Micronutrients   176
The Healthy Eating Plate   177
Vegetables & Fruits   180
Whole Grains   180
Protein   182
Water   183
How Much Water Do You Need?   185
Electrolytes   186
Caloric Intake   187
Sample Daily Menu   192
Summary   195

10. WARM UP, COOLDOWN AND RECOVERY   196
Warming Up & Cooling Down   196
Recovery   199

Conclusion   203
Exercise Appendix   211

BREAKING BAD EATING HABITS

Introduction 223

STEP ONE. IDENTIFYING HABITS

1. **PRE-BIRTH NUTRITION, PARENTAL AND SOCIETAL INFLUENCE** ... 231
   - Nutrition During Pregnancy 231
   - Childhood Influences 234
   - Media Influence 240
   - What About Eating Disorders? 242
   - Summary 243

2. **HOW BAD NUTRITION AFFECTS THE AGING PROCESS** ... 244
   - How the Body Changes As We Age 245
   - Changing Nutritional Needs 250
   - 9 Foods That Older People Need to Reduce 256
   - 9 Foods That Older People Need to Increase 261
   - Avoiding Weight Gain As You Age 265
   - Summary 266

3. **STRESS AND OUR GUTS** 269
   - Stress and Aging 271
   - The Effect of Stress on Your Gut 271
   - How Stress Affects the Digestive System 274
   - How Your Gut Bacteria Get Out of Balance 275
   - The Mood / Food Connection 278
   - Stress & Weight Gain 283
   - Stress & Thinking Ability 284
   - Stress' Impact on Metabolism 285
   - Top 10 Ways to Deal with Stress 285
   - Summary 298

4. **WHY DIETS DON'T WORK FOR MOST PEOPLE** 300
   - Why Diets Don't Work 304
   - Fad Diet Danger Signs 310

What About Intermittent Fasting? 313
Summary 314

STEP TWO. CHANGING MINDSET

5. IDENTIFYING THE RULES & HABITS WE NOW LIVE BY 319
   Mindful Eating 320
   Slowing Down: The Essence of Mindful Eating 325
   Identifying Your Eating Habits 329
   Analyze Your Eating Triggers 334
   Breaking Free from Binge Eating 340
   Breaking Free from the Binge-Restrict Cycle 346
   Summary 347

6. BREAKING THE RULES 349
   Issues of Self Esteem 350
   Understanding Hunger 353
   The TEN Types of Hunger 357
   3 Strategies for Adopting Healthy Eating Habits 361
   How Habits Work 363
   Changing a Bad Habit to a Good Habit 367
   A Dozen Nutritional Changes to Embrace Before You Turn 40 368
   Summary 370

STEP THREE. PRACTICAL SOLUTIONS

7. FUEL, HYDRATION & RECOVERY 375
   Spotlight on the Macronutrients 377
   The Importance of Sleep 385
   Summary 391

8. SO, WHAT SHOULD MY MEALS LOOK LIKE? 393
Plant-Based Foods: Vegetables, Whole Grains & Fruits 396
Healthy Protein 402
Healthy Oils 404
Guidelines on Sugar and Salt 406
Eating in Moderation 407
Recap of Key Recommendations: 407
Portion sizes 408
Summary 409

9. CHANGES TO MAKE IN MEALS, SNACKS AND DESSERTS 411
Breakfast 411
5 Great Breakfast Recipe Ideas 412
5 Great Lunch Ideas 418
Dinner 425
5 Great Dinner Ideas 429
10 Healthier Dessert Options 437
Make Your Own Protein Bars 438
The Smoothie Solution 441
3 Great Smoothie Recipes 444
Summary 446

Conclusion 447
References 457

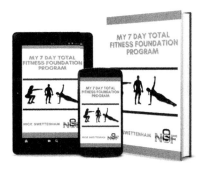

A Special Gift For My Readers

Included with the purchase of this book is My 7 Day Total Fitness Foundation Program to help you get started on your fitness journey. This program is a great way to start or adapt your training using all my 7 foundations.
Click the link below and let us know which email address you would like it delivered to.

www.nickswettenhamfitness.com

TOTAL FITNESS AFTER 40

THE 7 LIFE CHANGING FOUNDATIONS YOU NEED FOR STRENGTH, HEALTH AND MOTIVATION IN YOUR 40S, 50S, 60S AND BEYOND

INTRODUCTION

Help! Get me out of this body!

What's happening to me?

This is not what I signed up for.

If you've ever had those thoughts while standing naked in front of a mirror, you're hardly alone. The sad reality is that most people who are in their 40s, 50s and beyond are dissatisfied with their physical condition. Many of them are overweight, understrength and overwhelmed by aches and pains, chronic illness and plummeting energy levels.

In short, they are pretty pathetic imitations of what they used to be - and of what they should be.

If that's you, you need to know that growing weaker and less fit does not have to be your destiny as you age. You have it within your capacity to wake up every morning better, healthier and stronger than when you went to bed the night before. And that is true whether you're 27, 47, or 67.

Chronologically, age means nothing. In order to preserve your age, you need to preserve your physicality. And the time to start preserving it is now.

That's because, by the time you enter into your fourth decade, your body is beginning to show signs of wear and tear...

- Blood vessels lose their elasticity, making the heart work harder to pump blood around the body
- Muscles, joints and tendons lose strength and flexibility
- Testosterone production plummets
- The metabolism slows down

Society expects you to start going downhill as a result of these natural consequences of aging. After all, it's what everyone else does, right?

Once they hit 40, they get fat, lethargic, sick and decrepit. Every decade the downward spiral continues - then they die.

Is that the sort of future you want?

It doesn't have to be.

You see, there are a whole lot of people who have totally flipped that script. At 40, 50 and even 60 something they are genuinely in the best shape of their entire lives!

How have they done it?

By rejecting the ridiculously low bar that society has set for them and by learning the truth about fitness, health and well-being over 40.

That truth is what you will learn in this book.

It is encompassed within the 7 foundations that you must incorporate into your life in order to stay strong, lean and healthy at any age.

When you know, understand and apply the 7 foundations you will have the solution to the problems that plague many people in their 40s and beyond…

- Lost muscle and strength
- Decreased mobility and flexibility
- Lost confidence in their ability to train intensely

Your body does change when you age, and in this book, you will discover exactly how it does so. More importantly, though, you will find out precisely how you need to adjust your training to compensate for those changes.

This book will also show you how to infuse your mind with the mental strength to power you through the physical changes that will make you more powerful. By applying the strategies I'm about to share with you, you'll become laser-like in your ability to set, hone in on and systematically work toward the accomplishment of your goals.

Critically, we also demystify the whole subject of fitness nutrition. No other subject has led to such confusion, frustration and disappointment. Yet, what you eat is more important than anything else that you do. In Chapter Nine, you will finally learn how to eat the right way for your body.

Of course, there are literally thousands of books on getting in shape. So, why should you listen to what I've got to say?

Well, the honest answer is that you shouldn't. You should listen to the science of fitness, anatomy, biomechanics, kinesiology and nutrition. The great thing about science is that it is objective - it is not swayed by emotion, popularity, gimmicks or money making trends. All of that science is presented, disseminated and distilled in the chapters that follow. In fact, they form the basis of the 7 foundations that will underpin your future fitness program.

The problem with science, however, is that it is often presented by people who have no practical, on the ground experience in the discipline that it is applied to. And that's where I come in. You see, I am a personal fitness trainer who has used these 7 foundations to help hundreds of men and women over the age of 40 to regain their youthful vigor, transform their bodies and become stronger, more agile and healthier than when they were in their 20s and 30s.

I've written this book because I train people every day who, even before they're 40, are struggling with all 7 of these foundations. In the over 40 age-group, though, it is particularly challenging due to changes occurring in their bodies. I find that my clients have little to no knowledge of what is happening, and have either lost their confidence or have never gained it in the first place. I want this book to inspire people to take charge and start implementing these foundations into their workout routines.

I'm passionate about the health and fitness industry – it is a huge part of my life (both work and personal) and I love to help my clients improve their function and quality of life.

Are you ready to show the world, and yourself, that over 40 doesn't have to mean over the hill?

Great, let's get started!

1

AS WE AGE, WE CHANGE

WHAT'S HAPPENING TO MY BODY?

Over the past hundred years there has been a dramatic lengthening of the average human lifespan. For hundreds of years that average hovered around the 35 year mark. By 1900 it was up to around 50. Yet, between 1900 and 2000, it shot up to around 80. Currently the average life expectancy in the US is 78.99 years. Unfortunately, those extended years have not equated to improved health. In addition to the natural consequences of aging, many people in their 40s and beyond suffer from a range of lifestyle related illnesses that negatively affect their quality of life.

In this chapter, we consider the natural physiological changes that are a part of the aging process. We will then identify how the right type of exercise in conjunction with the 7 foundations of optimum health can counter these effects by keeping us stronger, more flexible, agile, coordinated and injury free as we age.

How Your Body Changes as You Age

Cardiovascular System Changes

As it ages, the heart becomes less efficient at pumping blood around the body. As a result, it has to work harder to keep the same quantity of blood moving around the system. At the same time, the blood vessels become less elastic and fatty deposits may build up on the walls of the arteries. As a result, the arteries become stiffer and blood pressure increases.

Bone Density Changes

From the age of 30 onwards, your bone density (having reached its peak) will begin to deteriorate. From that point onward, the bones will begin to shrink. The loss of density will make the bones weaker and more susceptible to fracture. The aging process also causes the vertebrae between the spinal discs to contract, making a person shorter. In fact, from the age of 40 onward, the average person will lose about half an inch in height every 10 years.

Muscle Changes

From around the age of 30, the natural process of aging results in muscle tissue loss. Both the quantity of muscle tissue and the number of muscle fibers are depleted. Fast twitch fibers deplete more so than slow twitch fibers, with the result that the muscles are slower to contract.

By the time they are 75, the average person will lose 25 percent of the muscle mass they had when they were 30. This muscle loss occurs more quickly in the lower part of the body than the upper part.

The reduction in the number of muscle fibers results in diminishing strength levels. This loss of strength, combined with the reduced balance that is another consequence of aging, may result in increased incidences of falling and losing one's balance.

Running in tandem with age related loss of muscle fibers, there is a corresponding loss of motor neurons. Shockingly, by the age of 60, the average person will have only 50 percent of the number of motor neurons they had when they were 20. These motor neurons are what control and drive muscle fiber activity. When they deplete, the muscle fiber will eventually die off.

The muscular system affects virtually every action that we take, so its weakening has profound effects on all areas of life. Age related muscle decline is known as sarcopenia. Its cumulative effect on body functioning shows difficulty in performing everyday tasks, such as carrying groceries, walking up flights of stairs or opening cans.

Hormonal Changes

We can think of hormones like orchestra conductors in that they control and regulate the myriad actions that are taking place in your body every second. Androgenic hormones are those that regulate male characteristics. The prime androgenic hormone is testosterone. Its main job is to regulate sexual functioning. Secondary functions include controlling muscle mass, strength levels, fat deposits and bone density.

Testosterone is well known as the key muscle building hormone. In fact, there is an out of control anabolic steroid market that allows people to inject synthetic versions of testosterone into their veins in order to get bigger and stronger. In addition to aiding the muscle mass increase, testosterone will also slow down muscle loss.

From around the age of 25, natural testosterone production begins to drop off. This age related testosterone decline speeds up when you enter your 30s, dropping by about 1 percent every decade. That's why it is harder for a guy in his 40s to build muscle than a guy in his 20s.

Even though it is a male sex hormone, testosterone is also important for women. That's because it is converted to estrogen (the female sex hormone) as well as promoting bone health, sex drive and fertility.

Testosterone is not the only hormone that diminishes as we age. Most of them do. Even with those that remain at constant levels, the decreased sensitivity of hormone receptors makes them less potent. In addition to testosterone, the key hormones which decline with age are estrogen, melatonin and growth hormone.

Melatonin is known as the sleep hormone. Its age-related decline is a key contributor to the sleep problems that so many people encounter as they age.

In men, the reduction of growth hormone combines with lower testosterone levels to further impact strength and muscle levels.

In women, the lowering of estrogen production is a direct contributor to menopause. This is characterized by the ending of menstruation. The levels of estrogen will fluctuate markedly in the years prior to and just after the onset of menopause. Bone density will decrease quite markedly after menopause. The onset of menopause is also accompanied by hot flashes.

The average age for the onset of menopause in women in America is 52, though it may commence from 45 years onward. Such lifestyle factors as smoking may cause an earlier onset of menopause.

Reduced levels of estrogen lead to other changes after the onset of menopause. These may include vaginal atrophy which makes sexual intercourse painful, thinning of the urinary tract that may make a woman more susceptible to urinary tract infections, and urinary incontinence. Lowered estrogen levels will also result in lowered levels of collagen and elasticity which reduces the elasticity of the skin.

Lower levels of estrogen will also exacerbate the age related decline in bone density. As a consequence of this, women will lose bone mass by about 5 percent more than men in the five years after the onset of menopause. It then levels off to be about the same rate as men.

Post menopause, women will also experience an increased level of LDL (bad) cholesterol, while the HDL (good) level remains the same. Women are also more prone to fat accumulation around the hips and waist after menopause.

Skin Changes

As we age, our skin becomes less elastic, thinner and drier. Fine wrinkles develop naturally but are made worse by long years of exposure to the sun. The main reason for these changes is the reduction in the levels of the fibrous tissue collagen and the flexible protein elastin. As well as making less of these compounds, aging actually changes their chemical structure so that they become less effective in keeping the skin looking young.

Another effect of aging on the skin is a thinning out of the fat layer directly under the skin. This takes away a layer of protection while also exacerbating the wrinkling effect of aging skin. The thinning of this fat layer also removes a means of insulation so that, as we age, we become less tolerant to the cold. At the same time, the body is less efficient at controlling heat. The number of sweat glands and blood vessels reduces with every passing decade. This makes it harder for heat to be moved from within to without the body. For this reason, older people are more likely to succumb to heatstroke.

A final effect of aging on the skin is that it is less able to absorb Vitamin D from the sun. That is why elderly people are more likely to have a Vitamin D deficiency.

Brain & Nervous System Changes

The brain changes more than any other part of the body as we grow older. From around the age of 30, the brain begins to shrink in size. Some areas of the brain get smaller faster than others. The three areas that are most affected are:

- The prefrontal cortex
- The cerebellum
- The hippocampus

It is interesting to note that these three areas are also the last to develop during adolescence. As a result, scientists have developed the last in, first out theory, by which the last parts of the brain to develop are the first parts to deteriorate.

As we age, the neurons in the brain get smaller in size and retract their dendrites. The number of synapses between the brain cells also diminishes, which has marked effects on brain functioning. Neurogenesis, or the creation of new neurons, also slows down with aging. Chemical messengers, including dopamine and serotonin, also become less frequent as we get older.

As a result of these changes in the brain, our memories become less effective, reflexes are slower, and coordination and balance are negatively impaired.

Urinary Tract Changes

Every decade beyond the age of 30, the kidneys become less effective at doing their job of eliminating waste from the body. Ten percent of people over the age of 65 experience a loss of bladder control. Urinary incontinence is more frequent in women than in men. This may occur as a result of the weakening of the sphincter muscles around the opening of the bladder. In men, it is caused by enlargement of the prostate.

Sleeping Pattern Changes

Contrary to what many people think, you do not need less sleep as you age. The reason that a lot of older people find it hard to get as much sleep as when they were younger is a combination of some of the factors we have already mentioned. This includes a lessening of the body's production of melatonin and a need to urinate more frequently.

Body Composition Changes

The natural loss of muscle tissue that occurs with aging is accompanied by most people with an increase in levels of body fat. A person's metabolism will naturally slow down as they age. This means that, even if they maintain the same caloric intake in their 50s as they did in their 30s, they burn fewer of them for energy and store more of them as body fat. In tandem with this is a general slowing down of activity as we age, meaning that we are burning off fewer calories.

From the age of 30 years onward, the average weight gain is around a pound a year. That may not sound like much. But between the ages of 30 and 60 that's an extra 30 pounds of weight that we're all lugging around!

Don't Worry, There's Good News Too!

After reading that litany of bad news, I wouldn't blame you if you're not feeling too optimistic about your physical future. Well, let me provide you with some good news ...

You can do something about it.

You may not be able to reverse all of the effects of aging, but you can most definitely do enough to reclaim the energy, vitality, strength and muscle mass that you thought were gone forever. The bottom line is that you can't stop the aging process, but you can most definitely slow it down.

The process by which you will be able to thrive into your 40s, 50s, 60s and beyond begins with a mental makeover. Rather than viewing each passing year as an excuse to do less, feel less and be less, take the opposite view. Consider the natural declines that occur with aging as a personal challenge. Make it your determination to, each day, be better than the day before. Rather than dreading your next birthday, welcome it. Embrace your age, determined to do whatever it takes to optimize your physical self.

In short, view the glass as half full rather than half empty!

WHAT FITNESS CAN DO FOR YOU

The key to thriving in your older years can be summed up in the word 'fitness'. However, fitness has come to be defined within narrow parameters in recent decades. In the next section, we will unpack what total fitness encompasses. For now, though, we can consider it to be the result of a lifestyle that prioritizes physical and mental well-being.

When you move beyond your 40th birthday, there are a number of lifestyle factors that should underpin your fitness lifestyle. Consider the following 7 factors and think about how you stack up in regard to them. Do you:

- Get regular (at least 6 monthly) medical checkups?
- Not smoke?
- Get regular exercise?
- Eat sensibly and in moderation?
- Strive to maintain a balanced weight?
- Know how to relax?
- Drink alcohol in moderation?

Even though I haven't gotten specific in terms of what regular exercise should look like or what constitutes healthy nutrition and balanced weight, I want you to give

Your fitness program will make you physically stronger. If you are new to resistance exercise, you should be able to improve your strength level by as much as 40 percent over a 12-month period. That will not only offset natural age-related strength decline, it will provide you with the power to accomplish the tasks that many people who age struggle with. At the same time, increased levels of physical strength add to the confidence that is the hallmark of a well-adjusted, healthy individual.

Along with your increased strength will come larger and tighter muscles. The changes that a few extra pounds of lean muscle tissue to a person's body composition makes can be quite dramatic. Adding some lean muscle to your shoulders, pectorals, back and quadriceps won't turn you into a bodybuilder but it will help you to sculpt the athletic type of physique that tells others that you care about your body and know how to look after it.

The more muscle you carry on your body, the less likely you will be to carry excess body fat. That's because muscle is very energy dependent. It takes about five times more energy to preserve an ounce of muscle than it does an ounce of fat. So, putting on muscle will speed up your metabolism, countering yet another of the natural effects of aging.

THE 7 FOUNDATIONS OF TOTAL FITNESS

The majority of people who work out put all of their energies into one particular form of fitness. For some it

yourself a rating out of 7 as to how you stack up against this list. If you are doing each of these things, give yourself a point. If not, don't.

Take a moment to think about how you score.

If you identify an area where you need work, that's ok. When you begin to put into practice the 7 foundations of total fitness, you will find it a lot a lot easier to make that change. For now, it's enough to realize that the need exists and you have the desire to do something about it.

So, what benefits will you get from taking on a total fitness program?

The benefits of fitness start on the inside and radiate outwards. After your first workout, you will begin to feel better about yourself. The fact that you are taking your health in your own hands will give you a feeling of control that is missing in many people's lives. Too often, people act as if their body is a runaway car that's out of control and heading for a cliff. Exercise allows you to slam on the brakes, throw the vehicle into reverse and then head back onto the freeway of life.

When you take control of your physical future in this way, you develop self-confidence. You'll begin to walk a little taller and prouder. After an exercise session, you will have a feeling of accomplishment. At the same time, feel good endorphins will flush through your body, producing a natural high that will set you up for a great day.

could be training with weights, while others spend the majority of their workout time in the cardio area or pounding the pavement as distance runners. However, the combination of decades of research and in the trenches experience has made it abundantly clear that the anti-aging benefits of fitness require a holistic approach to exercise.

A holistic approach means giving equal emphasis to each of the following 7 types of fitness:

1. Strength
2. Flexibility
3. Mobility
4. Stability
5. Agility
6. Endurance
7. Nutrition

These 7 foundations of total fitness can be considered a pension for your body and future function. The more you put into it, the more you get back!

Let's drill down on these foundations, one by one...

Strength

We haven't traditionally associated strength training with seniors. Yet, increasing the strength of the skeletal muscles has been shown to be profoundly beneficial as we age. In the past, the few seniors who discovered the benefits of strength training did so as part of their rehab program after an injury or accident. We now know that proactively beginning a strength training program in your 40s or 50s can help prevent those accidents or injuries from occurring in the first place.

Studies conducted over the past decade have shown that regular strength training can significantly reduce the symptoms of the following age - related conditions:

- Arthritis
- Poor balance
- Diabetes
- Osteoporosis
- Obesity
- Back pain
- Breathing problems
- Depression
- Dementia

In addition to making you far less likely to suffer from these and other health conditions, strength training will make you far more functional in your everyday tasks. A meta study out of the Department of Occupational Therapy at Indiana University-Purdue University Indianapolis analyzed 121 trials involving 6,700 study participants between the ages of 60 and 80. The researchers concluded that seniors who participated in strength training workouts two to three times per week consistently outperformed those who didn't on common daily movements.

Strength training has been shown to improve emotional makeup and to promote better sleep. It also builds self-esteem and self-efficacy. Researchers are still trying to determine the reasons why strength training has such a positive powerful effect on the mind yet are unanimous that it is as effective as medication at relieving depression.

Flexibility

Flexibility is the ability of your muscles, ligaments and tendons to elongate to their maximum potential. Flexible muscles are stretchy and pliable.

If you don't have good flexibility, such everyday activities as getting out of bed, bending down to pick up a child or squatting down to lift a heavy object can become more demanding. A lack of adequate flexibility can also impair your athletic ability, as you will be unable to reach the full potential, strength and power of your muscles.

Flexibility Benefits

Increased Range of Motion: Range of motion is the distance and direction your joints can move. Consistent flexibility training will increase the range of motion of your joints and muscles. It does this by lengthening the muscles and opening the joints. As a result, you'll be able to stretch further in all directions while remaining pain free.

Decreased Risk of Injury: People with flexible muscles are less likely to become injured during physical activity.

Reduced Muscle Soreness: Flexibility training helps to reduce muscle soreness after you exercise. When you stretch after your workout, you keep your muscles loose and relaxed.

Mobility

Mobility is strength through the full range of motion of an exercise. Unlike flexibility, it relies on the muscle alone to produce the range of movement. So, a flexible person may be able to raise his straightened leg quite high with the assistance of their arm. A mobile person, however, will be able to manipulate their leg or other muscle without any help at all.

Many people who focus exclusively on strength training are strong through a limited range of a muscle's motion. Others are very mobile in parts of the body but not in others. We can think of cyclists with well-developed and mobile legs but poor development and mobility in the upper body.

Total fitness requires balanced mobility throughout the whole body.

Stability

By the time you reach the age of 40 you will very likely have developed a number of muscular imbalances throughout your body. This is the result of decades of doing the same actions over and over again. For many people, this is seen as a propensity to lean forward, hunch over and carry themselves with extremely poor posture. The result is muscular imbalance and instability.

When our body is unstable, some muscles are stronger and more flexible than others. We develop what are referred to as overactive and underactive muscles. The over reliance on our overactive muscles makes the imbalance worse every day. It not only robs us of our stability and balance but sets us up for injury.

Stability training focuses on how to stabilize the body and how to move correctly. It prepares a person to react with optimized reflexes to any situation while maintaining proper joint alignment.

Agility

Agility is the ability to move, not only freely and easily but also quickly and gracefully. Being agile means you can feel fitter and more vibrant than ever before! Agility training is vital for professional athletes to perform at a high level but also for everyday folk as well. Regular agility training will lead to enhanced speed and alertness.

There is no better form of exercise to enhance your balance and coordination than agility training. Agility exercises will also help you develop greater eye - hand and foot coordination and help prevent other injuries. As you will discover later in this book, agility training can also be a lot of fun!

Endurance

Muscular endurance relates to the body's ability to exert force over a period of time. It is the difference between being able to do a one repetition squat with a maximum weight and the ability to maintain the wall sit position for 10 minutes. The squat demonstrates the strength of your quadriceps while the wall sit reveals the endurance of that muscle.

Muscular endurance is closely linked to the concept of physical stamina - the ability to sustain an activity for a prolonged period. The more stamina you have, the greater your ability will be to carry out such everyday tasks as washing your car or raking up the leaves in your yard. You'll be able to continue an activity without feeling fatigued or exhausted. And when the grandkids come over, you will have the energy to get active with them without feeling like you need respirator relief after they've gone.

Muscular endurance training, in which you use a lighter load for higher repetitions, will increase the health of your bones and joints. The reduced likelihood of muscular fatigue will also lessen your likelihood of suffering a fatigue related injury or accident.

Cardiovascular endurance is another vital aspect of total fitness. It will help you to sustain aerobic exercise and is an indication of the health of your heart and lungs. The more cardiovascular endurance you have, the more efficiently your heart is able to pump oxygenated blood to your muscles.

Nutrition

Your body is made from the nutrients contained in food:

- Water
- Protein
- Carbohydrate
- Fat
- Vitamins
- Minerals

Nutrition is the science of how our bodies utilize food. It boils down to two things:

1. Food's ability to produce energy to allow us to function
2. The nutrients we need to build, maintain and repair the organs and systems in our bodies.

When you put 'unhealthy' foods into your mouth day after day, your body will eventually start to suffer. This can lead to numerous health issues that we will explore in chapter nine.

Everyone has their own idea of what constitutes good nutrition. We just need to look at the wide disparity among diet types to confirm this. They run the full spectrum from zero carbs to zero fat and back again. It's no wonder that so many people are so confused when it comes to just what to put into their mouths to promote health and fitness!

When thinking about your nutrition, it is helpful to understand the four important criteria that all good nutrition plans must meet. They must:

- Control energy balance
- Provide nutrient density
- Achieve healthy body composition
- Be outcome based

While other factors, such as exercise, sleep and lifestyle habits all affect our health and wellness, their effect is minimal in comparison to nutrition. That's why we all need to apply the four basic criteria of nutrition in order to provide our bodies with the fuel that it needs to operate optimally.

KEY POINTS

- As you age, your body naturally becomes less efficient. Changes you will go through include losing muscle mass, slowing of your metabolism, and producing less testosterone.
- You have the power, through exercise, to slow down the aging process.
- Exercise will improve your self - image and your self-confidence.

- Regular exercise will make you physically and mentally stronger, improve your bone strength, body composition, coordination and balance.
- Exercise will boost the efficiency of your heart and lungs and make you far less likely to succumb to age-related disease.
- The 7 foundations of total fitness are strength, mobility, flexibility, stability, agility, endurance and nutrition.

2

DEVELOPING A MINDSET FOR SUCCESS

Every action you take begins with a thought. When it comes to making changes to your physical health, the way you think about yourself and about the world at large is critical to your success or failure. Unless you get your mind primed for success, you will fail to achieve your goals, regardless of what else you do.

We are living in an out of control world. People are so busy nowadays that they hardly have time to think - let alone breathe - before they're off to the next appointment, the next pick up or the next thing on their to do list. As a result, many people accept what happens to them as inevitable, as something over which they have little control, or as pure chance. They pile on weight, fail to stick to an exercise program or ditch their clean eating plan when the pressure comes on like waves that are being tossed about in an ocean of ill-disciplined self-indulgence and mediocrity.

The truth is very different. Every person - me and you included - has the power to take control of their destiny. We are not controlled by circumstance, unless we choose to be. This is especially so when it comes to the most personal and precious thing we possess - our health.

A balanced life, one in which we are giving proper attention to maintaining our physical, emotional, spiritual and psychological health, is within the grasp of each one of us. All we need is the courage to reach out and grasp hold of it.

Often the roots of people's inability to find success is rooted in negative self-talk. We are talking to ourselves all day long - you're probably doing it as you read these words. In fact, on the average day, you think some 60,000 thoughts. The majority of them are repetitive. Now for the startling part – most people's inner talk is predominantly negative. As a result, they are constantly feeding themselves with pessimism. They tell themselves 'I'll always be fat', 'It'll never work for me because I love food too much', or 'I can't do that'.

Learning to reprogram our minds to eliminate negativity is fundamental to taking control of our physical destiny. Spend the time to do that and everything else - the physical things like exercising and eating - will be so deeply ingrained in your psyche that you will be programmed for success. A lean, supple, energetic body will soon follow.

To think about...

What is the state of your inner self talk? Over the next 24 hours, consciously track your inner dialogue to gauge how many thoughts are couched in negativity. Whenever you catch one, kick it out and replace it with a positive affirmation.

Here are four more strategies to overcome negative self-talk:

- Question your thinking; before condemning yourself when you slip up, pause and question your thinking. If it's irrational, dismiss it!
- Eliminate self-prejudice; self-prejudice causes us to distort reality. To counter it, try to judge yourself as if you were an impartial observer.
- Own your imperfections; stop expecting perfection from yourself. Accept your faults and move on.
- Build your self-esteem; engage in new and different activities, such as playing sports and exercising.

THE POWER OF VISUALIZATION

A major key to achieving success is the ability to plant in the forefront of your mind vivid imagery of yourself successfully doing the thing that you want to achieve. A few years ago, mental imagery, also known as visualization, was the domain of professional athletes and self-help gurus. In recent times, however, there has been an increasing appreciation for the positive effects of mental imagery on goal attainment among the everyday exerciser.

When you regularly visualize yourself accomplishing your goals in your 'mind's eye', you provide a powerful stimulus to success. All you need to do is to utilize your imagination and focus to mentally rehearse the attainment of your goals. Start at the daily level and do it while you are lying in bed before you get up in the morning. See yourself doing everything that you need to in order to have a perfect goal attainment day, from springing out of bed, enjoying a healthy nutritious breakfast, powering through an invigorating, calorie depleting work-out and then enjoying an energy restoring post work-out shake.

When you're lying in bed at night, you should undertake another mental imagery session. See yourself having accomplished your end goal with the body, the strength and the energy that you are working towards. Create a crystal-clear image of this new you and embrace the feelings that go with it – the self-confidence, the energy and the joy of accomplishment.

SMART GOAL SETTING

Most of us aren't very good at setting goals. Fortunately, an excellent template has been devised to help us get it right. It is summed up in the acronym SMART, which stands for:

- Specific
- Measurable
- Achievable
- Realistic
- Time Bound

Let's consider them one by one . . .

Specific

Your goals need to be specifically defined. If your goal is generalized, it will be impossible to know when you have achieved it. That is why your goal needs to have an element of detail. So, rather than setting the goal that you want to 'get fit', drill down to a specific goal like 'running a half marathon'.

Note, too, that it is always best to couch your goal in concrete, definite rather than hopeful terminology. So, rather than saying "My goal is to run a half marathon", rephrase it as "I will run a half marathon."

Measurable

As well as being specific, your goals also need to be quantifiable. That is why losing weight is not a goal. Unless you quantify the amount of weight you want to lose, you will never know when you get there. So, here again, you need to drill down. State how much weight you are going to lose or, even better, what body fat percentage you are going to achieve. That way you will be able to monitor your progress and know if you are on track to the goal's achievement.

Achievable

It's great to aim for the stars, but aiming for another galaxy is to merely set yourself up for failure. There is a definite link between achievable goals, realistic timelines and stepping stone goals. In this regard, there is no better example than Arnold Schwarzenegger.

As a teenager living in Thal, Austria, Arnold set goals that everyone who he told them to thought were ridiculous; to become the best built man in the world and then become a famous Hollywood movie star. Even the idea of getting to America was as distant as traveling to the moon for rural Austrians in the 1950s. Yet, Arnold had the ability to break down his major long-term goals into smaller goals, each of which fed into the next goal. In fact, he was able to break down his goals to such an extent that his daily actions, everything he ate and every rep he performed in the gym, were connected with the fulfillment of his major goal. That fueled his desire to steadily work toward the fulfillment of goals that, on their face, appeared to be unachievable.

Realistic

A realistic goal is one that you are actually able to achieve. If you are in your forties, your goal to become a fighter pilot is probably not going to happen. Instead, modify your goal to something that is more realistic, like learning to become a pilot and flying a private plane. If you are a natural weight trainer, and you're not six foot five, you are not going to end up with 24-inch biceps, no matter how many sets of curls you do! But you will be able to develop an extremely impressive set of guns in the mid to late teens.

Time Bound

We've already touched upon the importance of time in relation to your goals in terms of keeping the goal achievable. So, while you shouldn't set yourself up for failure by having an unrealistic timeline, it is vital that you do have some sort of time element to your goal. Without a timeframe, you do not have a goal at all, only a vague ambition. But with one, you have a deadline. As a result, your sense of urgency increases and you are more likely to attain your goal.

Write your goal like this . . .

It is 1st May and I have just completed a half marathon

Writing your goal in the first-person present tense is very powerful. By re-reading that goal several times daily you will be transmitting the message to your subconscious, where it will go to work to fuel your drive to succeed!

LEARNING TO LOVE EXERCISE

Most people view exercise as a means to an end. Most of them don't enjoy the experience. To them, exercise is like bad tasting medicine that they must take in order to protect their health. The sooner they get it over with, the better. If you have that viewpoint, you will never succeed in achieving your fitness goals.

Here are four keys to learning to love exercise.

Forget the Past

Over 70% of Americans are either sedentary or not receiving the minimum amount of recommended exercise. Despite knowing that they should be working out, a lot of these people simply don't like exercise. This attitude is typically formed very early on in life.

By putting aside the bad experiences you have had in the past and focusing on new things that you find enjoyable, you'll be able to make your mind over. The key is to find an activity that you really enjoy doing and use it as the foundation for your exercise session.

Pace Yourself

When you first start working out, don't go full out straight away. If you exhaust yourself straight off the bat, you'll be adding fuel to the idea that you don't like exercising. Take it steady and build up gradually, enjoying the training along the way.

Exercise is movement. It's not confined to the gym or a set block of workout time. It could be walking, swimming, playing basketball or any other activity that you enjoy that will get your heart rate up for 30 minutes.

Ditch the Excuses

A lot of people tell themselves that they don't have time for exercise. We're all incredibly busy with more and more demands coming in on us all the time. But exercise needs to be a priority in your schedule. It is, after all, the key to everything else. Unless your body is maintained you will not be able to do all of those other things that are tugging at your time. For that reason you must schedule your workout into your calendar as non-negotiable 'you' time. Let people know that you are not available during those times.

Sometimes we have excellent intentions to exercise, but simply can't build up the motivation. The key, again, is to find something that you enjoy doing. If you enjoy it, motivation will not be a problem. A great way to overcome lack of motivation is to ask a friend to be your workout buddy. If you know that someone is waiting for you, you're much more likely to turn up at the exercise venue than if you're just relying on your own motivation level to get you there.

A trap that people often fall into is to put barriers in front of their ability to exercise. They do this by telling themselves that they must buy something before they can begin. It could be new shoes, gym clothes or a stopwatch that they have told themselves they need before they can start training. These are really just ways to procrastinate.

The reality is that you don't need any special equipment in order to get started on an exercise routine. Put the excuses aside, save your money, and just get started.

Overcome Insecurities

A lot of people feel very self-conscious when it comes to exercise. They can easily let their own personal insecurities hold them back. They'll convince themselves that others will laugh at them. That is almost certainly not going to be the case. If you've felt these insecurities, you simply have to put aside what you think other people might be thinking and just go ahead and do the things that you've always wanted to do.

BUILDING THE EXERCISE HABIT

It's been said that habits are like a warm bath on a cold night – easy to get into, and hard to get out of. While that may be true of bad habits, many people find it extremely difficult to get started with good habits – and then to stick with them. However, by breaking down the latest research on habit formation we can identify a simple three step process which will allow anyone to cultivate new habits.

Researchers at the Massachusetts Institute of Technology have done a lot of research on habits. They have broken down the process of habit formation into three key steps which they call the habit loop. These three parts are . . .

1. Cue, which is the trigger that starts the habit
2. Routine, which is the habit itself
3. Reward, which is the benefit you get from doing the habit

Habits will not be formed without cues. This is true of both good and bad habits. So, we need to work hard to trigger the right sort of cues – those that will lead to our good habits and not our bad habits. When it comes to cues there are four main types – location, time, the actions of others and the action that you took immediately prior to starting the habit. Let's take a quick look at each of them.

Location is a major habit driver. Many habits are nothing more than responses to our environment. You can manipulate your environment to help develop your new habit. Let's say your desired new habit is to start going to the gym in the morning before work. Your key environment is your bedroom. Set it up to make it easy to get out the door rather than staying in bed. Lay out your gym clothes, have your trainers out and ready to slip on and place your gym bag by the front door.

Time cues are very common. We become conditioned to automatically do things at certain times of the day. We can use this to our advantage to trigger new habits. Tie your new habit to a time and day. Let's say that your new habit is to go to the gym three mornings a week before work. So, if it's Monday at 6:00 am, that triggers you to get up and get moving. It doesn't matter how you're feeling or what you'd rather do, it's automatic!

The actions of others are powerful influences on our habits. But recent research has shown just how pervasive that influence is. One study, published in the New England Journal of Medicine, revealed that people who have an obese friend are 57 percent more likely to become obese themselves. So, it is vital that you surround yourself with people who will support your habit. With our morning gym habit, it is a great idea to find a workout buddy, and to have people at work and home who ask about how your workouts are going and give you encouragement to keep it up. Getting a text from your friend at 6:10 in the morning to wish you well on your workout is a powerful incentive to make it happen.

The action you take immediately prior to the habit action is very important. The experts call this habit stacking. This is when you pair a desired new habit with another one which you have already mastered. Let's go back to the early morning gym habit. You may have already developed the habit of having a coffee first thing in the morning. Pair this with grabbing your workout bag. Write this down as an affirmation this way...

As soon as I've had my morning coffee, I'll grab my workout bag and leave the house.

Notice that the action cue is very specific. 'As soon as' leaves no room for wishy washiness.

The second phase of the habit loop is the actual performance of the habit. To help make it stick you should do it the same way and with the same rituals every time. We all have little rituals we perform before we do things. In the gym example, it could be the way that you set yourself before doing a squat, or the number of breaths you take before you lift the bar off the rack. You should also perform your habit in the same place every time.

The third and final phase of the habit loop is the reward. This is based on the scientific principle of operant conditioning. This states that if you get a good feeling after you do a habit, you will continue to do it. The types of rewards that we give to ourselves are individual. Just provide yourself with a small celebration every time you perform your habit. This could be as simple as crossing off your gym visits on a calendar over a period of a week, or month. Then, at the end of that time period you might purchase that book you've been wanting or go out for a restaurant meal. You don't have to continue to reward yourself extrinsically forever. Once the habit is established, your rewards will become intrinsic. For example, going back to our workout example, the endorphin rush, self-esteem and bodily improvements that you experience will be rewards in themselves.

Developing a new habit, it has been often said, takes 21 days. Yet, there is no science behind that number. For some it will become habitual sooner than that, for others it will take more time. Rather than focusing on a number, like 21 days, just focus on repeating the habit loop until you don't even have to think about it.

So, how do you stick to a new habit? The first way is to develop new habits one at a time. Make a list of all of the new habits you want to develop, then prioritize them. Start with the most important and focus exclusively on implementing that habit before moving to the next one. Another important tip is to break your habit down into mini-habits. With the gym example, we've already identified some key mini habits – setting out your gym clothes and getting your bag ready the night before, mixing up your pre-workout drink, doing your warm-up. Focus on doing those things and the rest will follow.

Creating the Ideal Workout Program

Now that you know how to cement in your new exercise habit, let's talk about creating the ideal program in order to maximize your workout time while ensuring proper recovery and covering all areas of fitness.

The FITT Principle helps us to achieve those goals. FITT stands for:

- Frequency
- Intensity
- Time
- Type

Frequency

The starting point to constructing your workout program is deciding how often you will exercise. The current general recommendations for physical activity are 150 minutes of aerobic activity week at moderate-intensity exercise. That equates to about half an hour a day, five days a week. That activity should include doing a range of physical activities that incorporate fitness, strength, balance and flexibility. However, such activities as gardening and playing sport should also be included in your total exercise count. Including these types of activities will help to make sure that you are getting the proper balance between exercise and recovery.

Alternatively, it is recommended that you do 75 minutes of vigorous intensity exercise on a weekly basis. On top of that, you should do muscle strengthening activity on at least two days per week.

Intensity

Intensity relates to how hard your workout is. Your intensity level depends on the type of exercise you are doing and your training goal. Intensity depends on your current fitness level and your skill level. You can adjust the intensity level of your workout by:

- Changing the resistance amount
- Adjusting the number of sets and repetitions
- Varying the cadence of movement
- Changing the rest time between sets and exercises
- Performing intensity enhancing techniques such as supersets, drop sets and pre-exhaustion training

Time

Time relates to the amount of time that you are investing into your training sessions. When it comes to cardiovascular exercise, the general guidelines recommend doing between 20 and 60 minutes. However, this will depend on the intensity of the exercise you are doing. Steady state low intensity cardio, such as walking on a treadmill, can be done for up to an hour at a time. In contrast, high intensity interval training (HIIT), which involves short sprints followed by even shorter rest intervals, should only last for a maximum of 20 minutes.

Varying the length and intensity of your cardio workouts will promote total fitness.

Strength training workouts will usually last between 30 and 60 minutes, depending on whether you are training designated body parts or your whole body.

Type

There are many different types of exercise that you can do to work the various elements that comprise total fitness. However, all of them can be divided into two broad categories

- Aerobic
- Anaerobic

Aerobic

Aerobic exercise primarily benefits the cardiovascular system. It strengthens the heart and lungs while, at the same time, burning off excess calories. Examples of aerobic exercise are walking, cycling and skipping.

The word aerobic means 'with oxygen'. When you perform aerobic exercise, your muscles are getting enough oxygen to produce the required energy. This type of exercise is done at a steady, moderate pace and can be sustained for a long period of time.

Aerobic exercise primarily uses slow twitch muscle fibers and is best for cardiovascular health and endurance training.

Anaerobic

Anaerobic exercise is high intensity, short duration exercise that you cannot keep up for a long time. Weight lifting and sprinting are examples of anaerobic exercise. The word anaerobic means 'without oxygen.' With this type of exercise, the oxygen demands on your muscles are greater than the oxygen supply. This results in the production of lactate and the stopping of the exercise.

Anaerobic exercise is best to work your musculoskeletal system.

The FITT Principle will help you to continue training at optimal effectiveness over time. You should begin your exercise habit with a light frequency, low intensity workout, relatively short time per session and two types of exercise (one aerobic and the other anaerobic). An example would be to walk three times per week for 30 minutes each time and to accompany this with two full body strength training sessions.

As your body adapts to your training, you need to adjust your workouts in order to place increasing demands on your body. If you keep doing the same things, month in and month out, your body will have no reason to respond by getting fitter and stronger. When you decide that you need to adjust your workout, you should change one or more of the elements of FITT. For example, you could:

- Increase the frequency of walking to 5 days; or
- Increase the intensity by speed walking; or
- Increase the time by walking for 45 minutes per session; or
- Changing the exercise type by cycling.

To be safe, you should only change one thing at a time. Once you have done a week or so of the adjusted workout, you can change another aspect to progress your fitness.

ENERGY SYSTEMS

Every breath you take, every move you make and every thought you think requires energy. When you work out, it needs it more than when you are at rest. All of the energy that allows you to function comes from the food that you eat. That food is broken down in the body to produce energy in the form of ATP (adenosine triphosphate).

ATP is stored in our muscle cells, but only in very limited amounts. That stored ATP will only supply the energy you need to exercise for a matter of seconds. To continue to function, the cells then require more ATP being made by the body.

There are three systems that the body can use to produce ATP:

- The ATP-PCR system
- The glycolytic system
- The oxidative system

The ATP-PCR and the glycolytic system are both anaerobic because they do not require oxygen. The oxidative system does require oxygen to make ATP.

The ATP-PCR system allows for exercise between 5-15 seconds. The ATP stored in the muscle will power up to the first five seconds. The salt phosphate (PCR) attaches to ATP to provide another 10 seconds or so of energy.

Once the ATP-PCR system is used up, the body switches to the glycolytic system. Now the body relies upon glycogen, which is the broken-down form of carbohydrate, to make ATP. This is achieved through the process of glycolysis. During glycolysis, lactate is produced, along with hydrogen ions. These are responsible for the muscle burn and fatigue you feel when sprinting or lifting heavy weights.

The glycolytic system will sustain you for up to two minutes of exercise. After that, the body switches to the oxidative system. With this system, ATP is produced using two mechanisms:

- The Krebs cycle
- The electron transport chain

The oxidative system produces ATP more slowly than the other two systems, but it will provide energy for a greater duration. This explains why you can run slowly for a long period of time, but sprint for only a short period of time, before you are exhausted.

It is possible to exercise each of the energy systems to be more efficient. Doing explosive plyometric moves like box jumps will improve your ATP-PCR system. Circuit training, where you move from one exercise to the next with little to no rest, will make your glycolytic system more efficient, and performing 20-30 minute cardio sessions of moderate intensity, such as walking, jogging or biking, can improve your oxidative system.

THE IMPORTANCE OF YOUR TRAINING HEART RATE

Zone heart rate training is based on exercise intensity and heart rate zones. There are five heart rate zones that are each based upon a person's maximum heart rate. While it is impossible to precisely work out your maximum heart rate, there are a number of formulas to provide you with a close estimate. The most common formula for working out your maximum heart rate is to subtract your heart rate from 220.

So, if you are 40 years of age, your max heart rate is . . .

$$220 - 40 = 180$$

Here's an overview of the 5 heart rate training zones . . .

Zone One

The first training heart rate zone represents a light intensity of training, such as going for an evening walk. This training heart rate zone is 50-60% of your max heart rate.

For our 40 year old exerciser, Zone One would be between 90 and 108 beats per minute.

Zone Two

The second training zone represents a medium intensity level, such as jogging or rollerblading. This training heart rate is 60-70% of your max heart rate.

For our 40 year old exerciser, Zone Two would be between 108 and 126 beats per minute.

Zone Three

The third training zone represents a light to medium intensity level, such as power walking and cycling. This training heart rate is 70-80% of your max heart rate.

For our 40 year old exerciser, Zone Three would be between 126 and 144 beats per minute.

Zone Four

The fourth training zone represents a high intensity level, such as sprinting and uphill cycling. This training heart rate is 80-90% of your max heart rate.

For our 40 year old exerciser, Zone Four would be between 144 and 162 beats per minute.

Beginner exercisers should not train in Zone 4 until they have built up their aerobic fitness level with around six months of training.

Zone Five

The fifth training zone represents your maximum heart rate. This is where your heart, lungs and respiratory functioning are all operating at full capacity. Only athletes who are at an extremely high level of fitness should train at their maximum heart rate. Examples of training at Zone 5 include Tabata style High Intensity Interval Training (HIIT). Zone 5 represents 90-100% of your maximum heart rate. For our 40 year old exerciser, Zone 5 would be between 162 and 180 beats per minute.

Keep in mind that the calculation for your max heart rate is just an estimate, so there is some margin of error. Over time, as you train more, your exercise intensity may have to change for each of the zones. For example, beginner exercisers who go for a light jog may be in Zone 3. But, as they continue to work out, their body will adapt and their fitness improves, so that in three to five weeks that same jog will only put them in Zone 2. That means that you have significantly improved your aerobic fitness level. Using a heart rate monitor is an easy way to track the heart rate zone you are working in, and your improvements in aerobic fitness over time.

KEY POINTS

- You have the power to be the master of your physical destiny
- Eliminate negative self-talk
- Use visualization to enforce your positive mindset
- Create SMART goals that are specific, measurable, achievable, realistic and time bound
- Learn to love exercise by forgetting the past, pacing yourself, ditching excuses and overcoming insecurities
- Build the exercise habit with cues, routines and rewards

- Use the FITT Principle to create your ideal workout program
- Work through all three energy systems to achieve total fitness
- Vary your training heart rate zone for total cardiovascular fitness

3

STRENGTH - YOU ARE STRONGER THAN YOU KNOW!

I'd like to begin this chapter with a bold declarative statement...

No matter your age or ability now, you NEED to take up strength training and perform it consistently over the course of the rest of your life. It is never too late to start and, as soon as you do, your body and your mind will start to reap immediate benefits.

Now, let's find out why I can make such an unequivocal recommendation.

When we consider aging and the diseases of modern civilization, we find that almost all of them are related to muscle loss that occurs with aging, or sarcopenia. It has also been shown that reversal or improvement in these diseases is preceded by the reclaiming of muscle mass and strength. As a result, for some reason that is still not fully understood, muscle and strength seem to be the key to maintaining our health as we age.

The American Council of Aging have identified the following 10 biomarkers of health:

1. Muscle Mass
2. Strength
3. Bone Density
4. Bone Composition
5. Blood Lipids
6. Hemodynamics
7. Glucose Control
8. Aerobic Capacity
9. Gene Expression
10. Brain Factors

How many of those essential biomarkers of health do you think strength training benefits?

Even if regular strength training improved 2 or 3 of these areas, wouldn't you agree that it would be a worthwhile activity to engage in?

Well, the fact is that strength training will produce marked improvement in ALL of these areas. That is not only remarkable, but also unequalled by any other activity. And that is why strength training needs to form the foundation of your health and wellness lifestyle.

Let's drill down on each of these essential health biomarkers to see just how strength training can help.

Muscle Mass / Strength

As people get older, they become more likely to fall and lose their balance. In fact, in 2016, falls became the number one cause of traumatic death in people over the age of 65. The common perception is that the elderly are more prone to falling due to arthritis and stiffness. But that is not the case. It is actually related to the loss of muscle, and in particular a type of muscle called Type II fiber. This type of muscle fiber is capable of producing a lot of force suddenly. Yet, these fibers are the most prone to atrophy and strength loss when they are not used.

When your Type II fibers are strong and numerous, they act rapidly and strongly as a counter when you lean forward or go off balance in order to right your balance and prevent a fall. This happens without your conscious awareness. But when you lose the functionality of these Type II fibers, that counter doesn't kick in and you fall over.

Skeletal muscle is the largest and most active endocrine / immunogenic organ in the human body. Your muscles are constantly sending chemical signals out to all of the tissues of your body. Those signals are vital to the optimal functioning of those tissues. As a result, strength training has benefits far beyond those related specifically to muscle mass and strength.

So, how beneficial is strength training to the restoration of muscle mass and strength?

In one study, a 30 percent loss of strength that had accumulated over 12 years was restored with just one year of strength training. As incredible as that turnaround sounds, it is, in fact, a modest result! Most people, when they follow an optimized strength training program will actually be able to improve their strength levels by as much as 300 percent in a 12-month period.

Bone Density

It has been known for some time that strength training can dramatically improve bone density. It used to be thought that this was due to increased mechanical load and stress on the bone with this type of exercise, but now researchers have discovered that it is in fact due to myokine signaling. When they are being stressed through exercise, muscles send out a hormonal signal to bones that promotes increased strength. The good news is that this signaling is not proportionate to the load that is on the muscle, which means that you don't have to overload the muscle with very heavy weights to promote bone density improvement.

Body Composition

Our body tissues are in competition with each other for nutrients. Myokines that are released from skeletal muscle as a result of strength training stress force the body to prioritize lean muscle tissue in nutrient allocation. The nutrients available will flow toward preserving the muscle rather than body fat. Strength training induced myokine increase also enhances fatty acid uptake from your fat cells as well as promoting an increase in glucose uptake and a speeding up of your metabolism. It has also been shown to activate insulin signaling. This mimics the action of the hormone leptin, decreasing inflammation in your body.

Strength training has also been shown to increase the release of the myokine Interleukin 15 from muscle cells. This myokine signals your existing fat cells and triggers a chemical called uncoupling protein to convert white fat (which is essentially an energy storing depot and precursor of inflammation) into brown fat, which speeds up the action of the mitochondria in the cell to produce more energy and, therefore, burn off more fat.

Blood Lipids

When it comes to blood lipids, doctors typically measure total cholesterol, HDL (good) and LDL (bad) cholesterol. Strength training will raise your HDL and lower your LDL cholesterol levels. More importantly, though, it opposes inflammatory myokines and controls insulin sensitivity and serum insulin levels. This is a major preventative against cardiovascular disease, which, according to the Center for Disease Control and Prevention, is the leading cause of death in the USA today.

Hemodynamics

Hemodynamics is all to do with blood flow. This is an area where strength training really outshines aerobic or steady state exercise. Starling's Law of the Heart describes how the heart functions; our heart works in a similar way to our septic system. It works optimally if the volume on the input side equals the volume on the output side. So, the cardiac output out of the left side of your heart is directly proportional to the amount of blood that is delivered to the right side of the heart. In other words, if 500ml of blood comes in, then 500ml will go out.

Coronary arteries come off the base of aorta and supply blood flow to the heart. The blood that returns to your heart through the coronary arteries is very passive. All the blood below the level of your heart gets there through muscle contraction and a one-way valve network that pushes the blood back to the heart. The intense muscular contraction involved in strength training enhances venous blood flow to the right side of the heart, which increases the blood volume that is pumped in the heart. In harmony with Starling's Law, this also increases the volume of blood that is pumped out of the left side of the heart. This also has the benefit of enhancing the backwash, which floods the coronary arteries and determines coronary artery blood flow.

Furthermore, the stronger the muscles, the more intense the muscle contractions that shunt blood up to the heart and the greater the amount of blood that will be pumped around the body will be. Strength training also decreases blood pressure.

In these ways, strength training has proven to be hugely beneficial for people with coronary artery disease.

Blood Glucose Control

Skeletal muscle is the biggest glucose reservoir in the body. When you do high intensity strength training, you exhaust your muscle's glycogen stores. This demands improved insulin sensitivity and improved glucose transport into the working muscle cell. This is the opposite to the metabolic syndrome that happens when we eat a bad diet and become sedentary.

Aerobic Capacity

Aerobic metabolism happens in the mitochondria of our cells. But aerobic metabolism cannot happen without anaerobic metabolism delivering its substrate, pyruvate, to the cell. Yet anaerobic metabolism delivers pyruvate to the cell at a rate faster than aerobic metabolism can handle it. So, the only way to maximally improve aerobic capacity is by doing hard anaerobic exercise such as - you guessed it! - strength training, that delivers pyruvate as fast as it can be aerobically metabolized.

Gene Expression

A landmark study in 2007 led by Dr. Simon Melov of the University of Southern California found that resistance training reduces aging in skeletal muscle tissue. The researchers identified 176 genes related to aging that reverted back to youthful levels of expression after just 26 weeks of strength training.

This was the first scientific study to show that it is possible to reverse aging at the genetic level.

How?

With strength training!

Brain Factors

Brain derived neurotrophic factor (BDNF) is a myokine that is known as the memory myokine. BDNF is low in people with Alzheimer's, depression and obesity, and is an independent marker for morbidity. Strength training has been shown to increase BDNF levels. Scientists do not know just how the mechanism works, but it is clear that BDNF produced in skeletal muscles is able to cross the blood brain barrier and produce significant cognitive benefits.

What is Strength Training?

We've seen that strength training addresses all ten of the biomarkers of health. That makes it unequalled in its ability to produce health benefits, especially as we age. So, now that we know that strength training is something that you should be doing, let's take a look at just what strength training involves.

Strength can be thought of like an iceberg. The part of the iceberg that is above the water is like the external strength that is seen when a person performs heavy lifts like the bench press or a deadlift. But hiding under the water, the 90 percent of your strength that is not outwardly visible has to do with the functional strength of the person's muscles as they work together. Often people who are very strong in one area, such as pressing overhead, have developed weaknesses in other areas, such as the glutes, hamstrings or lower back. As a result, they leave themselves open to imbalance injuries. They are also more likely to develop abnormal patterns of movement that sees them favoring their stronger muscles. This is often seen with poor posture which can result in problems like lower back pain.

The strength that is developed in your muscles is underpinned by the other 6 foundations of total fitness:

- Flexibility
- Mobility
- Stability
- Agility
- Endurance
- Nutrition

Strength training involves lifting and lowering weight in a controlled manner. You begin with a slow, gradual upload of resistance and then you work to make progressive resistance as you continue onward. You need to be lifting slowly and smoothly with the intent of using the resistance to bring about a deep level of fatigue in the working muscle.

When you place a strength training demand on the body, you are asking the body to make an adaptation to become stronger and more muscular in order to meet the demand in future. In this way, strength training is a stimulus. The adaptation that it stimulates requires time, recuperation and nutrients.

THE STRENGTH TRAINING PYRAMID

The Strength Training Pyramid is a graphic representation of the factors that should go into a properly structured exercise program. Here's what the pyramid looks like...

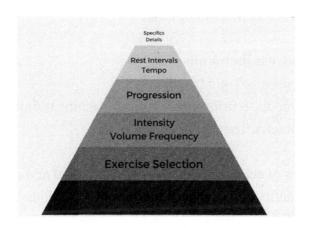

Let's consider the six levels of the Strength Pyramid one by one. At the bottom of the pyramid, we have Movement Quality.

MOVEMENT QUALITY

There are a number of different forms of exercise that you could do to improve your health. However, you only have a limited amount of time and energy to contribute to this part of your life. As a result, you need to select the form of movement that will give you the best bang for your buck - in other words, the quality of your exercise matters! For the reasons already presented in this chapter, if you had to produce just one form of exercise, that should be strength training.

But what sort of strength training should you do?

There are a number of options:

- Bodyweight training
- Resistance band training
- Dynamic tension free weight / machine training
- Isometric training

In terms of achieving the best biomechanical and anatomical benefits, the best form of strength training and the focus of this chapter is dynamic tension free weight and machine training. That is because dynamic tension strength training allows you to move a muscle through its complete biomechanical range of motion. As a result, the muscle lengthens and shortens to create muscle contraction following the natural strength curve of the muscle, which is hardest at the beginning of the exercise and easiest at the end of the exercise. You can also adjust free weights and resistance machines to a weight that is safe and suited to your strength on any given day.

In contrast, resistance band training reverses the natural strength curve, being easiest at the beginning and hardest at the end of the movement. If you do not have access to a gym or are going on holiday or a business trip, resistance bands are still a good alternative as they are small and easy to fit into a suitcase.

Isometric exercise does not move a muscle through its range of motion and instead involves static holds. This doesn't mean to say that they do not have significant benefits. They are still important for strength, muscle endurance, stability and involve the muscles to be constantly engaged during the exercise.

Bodyweight training is still very beneficial as it helps to improve strength, endurance, flexibility, balance and mobility. The problem with bodyweight training is that a lot of people simply do not have the strength to lift their own body weight. This can lead to very bad form and a high chance of injuries. For example: Sinking your pelvis during a press up due to a weak core can lead to lower back problems. A really handy piece of equipment to acquire is a suspension trainer. This can be used to aid bodyweight training exercises by controlling how much bodyweight resistance you use. Although not the focus of strength training in this book, I would highly recommend further looking into a suspension trainer.

NEXT UP IN THE PYRAMID IS EXERCISE SELECTION.

EXERCISE SELECTION

Correct selection of the exercises that you perform as part of your workout is critical in order to ensure that you are getting the maximum benefit from your training investment without causing injury to your body. Unfortunately, many of the exercises that are accepted as 'fundamental' to strength training do neither of those things. So, rather than simply doing what everyone else in the gym is doing, we need to approach the subject from an objective, scientific point of view.

There are a number of principles we can use based on biomechanical physics to rate how good an exercise is in terms of strength development and muscle stimulation. Here are 3 of them:

1. The exercise should allow the operating lever of the target muscle to move directly toward the origin of the muscle fiber. For example, the operating lever of a dumbbell curl is the forearm, and it moves toward the origin of the biceps which is the scapula.

2. The exercise should provide alignment between the direction of the resistance, the direction of the motion and the origin and insertion points of the muscle fiber. If we think about the latissimus dorsi muscle, the muscle fibers are mostly diagonal from their origin on the spine and their insertion on the upper inner part of the humerus (upper arm bone). Muscles always pull toward their origin, so the ideal movement for the lats is diagonally down from an angle where the arm is pulling at about 30 degrees down and in toward the hip. This is achieved with the One Arm Lat Pull In, rather than the Lat Pulldown, Chin Up or Seated Row, which are much more commonly seen in the gym, but none of which follow the direction of the muscle fibers.

Lat Pull In

1. The exercise should allow a muscle to move through its full range of motion. Let's consider the example of the deltoid (shoulder) muscles. There are three deltoid heads. The anterior (front) deltoid pulls the upper arm forward and upward. So its range of motion is from an arm position behind the torso and through to full arm extension in front of the body. The lateral (side) delts move the arms out to the side, while the posterior (rear) delt moves down and back. None of these ranges of motions look anything like what you are doing when you

perform the overhead press, which has traditionally been the 'go-to' exercise for the deltoids. The smart exerciser will choose exercises that follow the range of motion of the muscle in its natural movement.

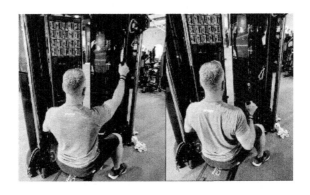

For the deltoids, those exercises are the following:

Cable Front Deltoid Press

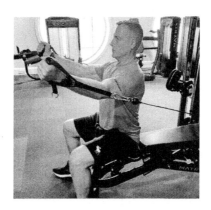

Rear Delt Cable Extension

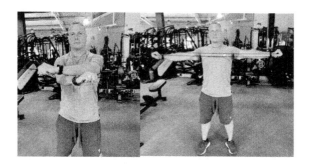

Cable Side Lateral Raise

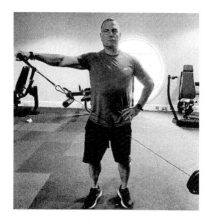

A lot of the exercises recommended later in this section have been selected because they follow these principles. Here are some examples of exercises that, although very common, do not align with the ideal principles outlined above. This compromises them in various ways. I'm not saying that you should never do these exercises, simply that there are more biomechanically beneficial options that come with a much reduced risk of injury as we age:

- Upright Rowing
- Preacher Barbell Curls
- Overhead Shoulder Press
- Barbell Squats
- Bent Over Barbell Row
- Barbell deadlifts
- Hanging Leg Raises

One reason the barbell deadlift can be so dangerous is that due to the bar being in front of your body, it forces your shoulders to protract forward, rounding the top of your spine. This also puts added load on your lower back. For an alternative, you can use what's known as a Hex or Trap bar. Your hands will now be at your sides which retracts the shoulders and engages your upper back more to take some of that load off the lower back. This will also engage the quadriceps more, but it's still a far safer option.

The next level in our strength training pyramid shows the importance of Intensity, Volume and Frequency.

INTENSITY, VOLUME, FREQUENCY

When you perform strength training exercises, you impose stress on the muscle. It is the adaptation to that stress that produces beneficial results. The reason that these adaptations occur is to prepare the muscle to meet that same stress level in future and be able to handle it. Unless your level of intensity is progressive, then you will not see a continual progression of benefits. That is because your body will already have adapted to the stress level.

Increasing the intensity of your workout can be achieved by increasing the resistance, increasing the time under tension (i.e. the amount of time you are contracting the muscle) or reducing the rest time between sets.

The volume of a strength training session relates to the total amount of work that you perform within a workout. It is possible to overtrain a muscle by doing too much just as it is possible to undertrain it by doing too little. The ideal volume for a muscle to elicit the maximum muscle building result seems to be 8-10 sets, with a rep range of between 6 and 20 reps. This wide rep range will allow you to stimulate all muscle fiber types, including Type II fiber, which we have already identified as being crucial in preventing falls and balance issues. You can also increase the volume of work by increasing your time under tension by taking longer to perform the movement, or adding isometric holds into each rep.

When designing our strength training program to achieve the correct intensity, volume and frequency, we need to consider metabolic stress. This describes the point when our muscles begin to fatigue, and we go into anaerobic metabolism. In this state, the muscles begin to accumulate lactate and other metabolites, and the muscle is infused with blood. Bodybuilders call this the 'pump'. This triggers protein synthesis and the subsequent building of new muscle tissue.

To achieve the desired level of metabolic stress, you need to include higher rep sets. Going up to 20 reps will achieve the pump effect needed. You can also achieve the peak contractions needed for maximum blood flow with isometrics.

Next up in the strength training pyramid is Progression.

PROGRESSION

To continue seeing benefits for your strength training investment, you need to be making the workout progressively harder. This can be done by:

- Increasing the resistance
- Increasing the repetitions

Let's say that you are doing the dumbbell curl with a weight that allows you to do 8 repetitions with good form. Each succeeding workout push yourself to perform an extra repetition without losing your good technique. When, after a period of weeks, you are able to do 12 reps with the weight that you started out doing 8 reps with, increase the weight slightly and drop back to 8 reps. You can continue progressing in this manner without limit.

Keep in mind that our strength can fluctuate for no apparent reason. Sometimes you may turn up for your workout and not be able to push past your previous limits. That's ok - so long as you are pushing yourself to the best of your ability on that day.

The penultimate level of the strength training pyramid considers rest intervals and tempo.

REST INTERVALS / TEMPO

The rest intervals between each set that you do should allow you to sufficiently recover from the previous set so that you are able to exert maximum force on the upcoming set. Of course, there will naturally be a cumulative muscle fatigue effect which cannot be avoided. You also want to build on the intensity of the last set to create a stair step stress effect on the muscle. All of this requires fine balancing of the ideal rest between sets time. Much research has gone into this subject. The consensus is that for maximum strength and muscle stimulation effect, you should rest for between 60-90 seconds per set.

Tempo relates to the speed with which you perform an exercise. You should perform your reps with a moderate tempo under control and without the use of any momentum.

A couple of factors that relate directly to your training tempo are time under tension and concentric / eccentric reps.

Time Under Tension

Time under tension, or TUT, refers to the total amount of time that a muscle is kept under tension in a set. When you incorporate TUT training in your workout, you prolong the time that your muscle is under tension in a rep by holding, or sometimes bouncing slightly, in the contracted position. TUT can also involve taking twice as long on the eccentric phase of the exercise than on the concentric phase. According to a 2016 study, doubling the length of the eccentric phase may result in greater muscle growth.

Concentric / Eccentric Reps

A repetition can be broken down into three parts; the lifting and the lowering portions, and the transition between them. The lifting part of the rep is known as the concentric, or positive, part, while the lowering portion is known as the eccentric or negative part.

Using the example of bicep curls, the lifting part where you curl the weight from your thighs to your shoulders is the concentric portion of the rep. The lowering part where you return to the start position is the eccentric portion. You are stronger during the eccentric part of the rep so that you can lower more weight than you can lift.

Research has shown that both the concentric and eccentric parts of the rep is beneficial to strength and muscle gains. You should take slightly longer on the eccentric part of the rep.

You should aim to follow a 2:1:3 tempo for best results. This means that you take 2 seconds to lift the weight (concentric), 1 second to hold in the peak contracted transition position and three seconds to lower the weight (eccentric).

A note on muscle damage - an effective muscle building workout will cause microtears in the muscle tissue. This will lead to soreness the next day and be the catalyst for protein synthesis. But we don't want to cause too much muscle damage, or all of the protein synthesis will go towards rebuilding old muscle rather than creating new muscle.

As you can handle a resistance that is as much as 20 percent heavier than you could on a concentric rep, when contracting your muscle concentrically, focusing on your eccentric reps is a great way to enhance muscle damage. You can also decrease the speed of the eccentric part of the rep, going from 2 to 4 seconds to complete the movement (i.e., increasing the TUT).

However, if you are focusing on eccentrics, the frequency of workouts must allow sufficient time for the muscles to recover from the stress imposed by your strength training session. Sufficient time is needed for the microtears in the muscle to repair themselves with the aid of the nutrients that you put into your body after the workout. That way they will grow back bigger and stronger than they were before your training session.

Finally, the apex of the strength training pyramid involves us thinking about the details of the program.

SPECIFICS/ DETAILS

The specifics and details relate to any customization of the program that are geared toward your specific goals and needs. For example, if you have a specific area of weakness, such as in the hamstrings, you might work them more than your quads in order to balance the strength between opposing muscle groups.

STRENGTH TRAINING IN PRACTICE

Society has fed us on the notion that older people have completely unique exercise requirements than younger people. That is completely false. Being older doesn't change much about your body's physiological needs for exercise. The muscles are still in the same place, they still have the same origin and insertion points, and they still respond in the same way to the stress of strength training.

The only difference between a 25-year-old and 55-year-old is that the 55-year old's body has had an extra 30 years to decondition itself. During this time, if he or she has not been doing strength training, his muscles will have atrophied. Yet, both the 25 and the 55-year-old require the same physiological mechanism to get stronger and build muscle. The 25-year-old and the 55-year-old both need to follow the same safety precautions, though the older person has a greater need to adhere to them.

All strength trainers need to perform biomechanically correct movements that allows them to move the muscle through a full range of motion. The exercise must also be done in such a way that it properly tracks joint and muscle function. The exercise must also be done in such a way that it properly controls the forces brought to bear on the muscles, joints and connective tissues.

One key issue to avoid at any age, but especially when you get past your 40th birthday, is excessive spinal loading. One of the main exercises in the gym that causes excessive spinal loading is the barbell squat. This exercise involves a tremendous amount of spinal compression due to the heavy weight that sits at the top of the spinal column. That load overloads the erector spinae and can cause irreparable disc damage. A far safer and wiser option, especially for older people, is to perform the cable or goblet version of the squat movement.

Perform the cable squat by setting a double pulley cable machine to its lowest pulley setting. Face the machine and grab the handles, stepping back about half a meter from the weight stacks so that your arms are fully extended. Try to stay upright as you squat down to a full squat position and then push through your heels to return to the start position. You will feel this movement directly working in the quadriceps, without compromising your spine.

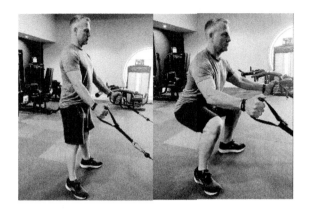

As an older exerciser, your focus needs to be on controlling the weight that you are using. That may require reducing the weight. Too many people, especially those who exercise in a commercial gym, work out to impress others or to achieve a certain weightlifting goal. That is not the way to get results. Never let the desire to go heavy get in the way of proper exercise form.

Keep in mind that your muscles have no idea what the number is on the side of the weight. All it knows is how much stress is being applied to it. Using a weight that is correct for your ability, you can control for the desired number of reps. This will place more stress on the muscle - and therefore generate more results - than a weight that is too heavy, requiring you to use momentum and the assistance of other muscle groups to get the weight up. By using lighter weight and slowly down the eccentric (negative) part of the movement you will be amazed at the results.

As an older trainer you should also focus on developing the mind muscle connection. Concentrate on how the muscle feels during the movement. See the muscle fibers expanding and contracting in your mind's eye and become attuned to the feel of that movement. This will allow you to get the maximum benefit out of every rep. It will also allow you to develop joint stability and muscle control.

When you were younger you may have emphasized working the 'show' muscles of the body, such as the biceps and chest, abs and glute muscles. As you get older, however, you need to train more wisely. That means not neglecting any of the major muscles of the body. Any body part that is neglected will become your weak link.

You need to be training each of the following body parts as equally as possible:

- Pectorals
- Latissimus Dorsi
- Deltoids
- Trapezius
- Rhomboids
- Rotator Cuff
- Biceps
- Triceps
- Forearms
- Abdominals and Obliques
- Erector Spinae

- Quadriceps
- Glutes
- Hamstrings
- Calves

SAMPLE WORKOUTS.

The following strength training workouts are designed for a person who has not done any regular strength training before or who is getting back into a resistance training routine. You will need access to a gym for these workouts. This is a two-day split, so that the person is training half the body one day and the other half of the body the next day. The emphasis for the first couple of workouts is to learn the proper exercise motion and establish the mind muscle connection that we have spoken about. You should also be experimenting to find the correct weight for the repetitions you are performing. From your third session onward, you should be working to increase the intensity of each workout by increasing the reps or the resistance.

On each successive set that you perform for an exercise, increase the weight slightly.

WARMING UP / COOLING DOWN

You must warm-up before every workout. Doing so will raise your body temperature, increase the mobility of your joints, increase blood flow and get you mentally primed.

Begin each workout with 3- 5 minutes of light cardio. If you don't have access to an exercise bike or treadmill, you can simply jog around your garden/ outdoor space. Or jog on the spot for 60 seconds, perform jumping jacks for 30 seconds, followed by high knees for another 30 seconds and repeat 2-3 times.

Next, do some dynamic stretching specifically to the body parts you will be working on. These could include arm circles, leg swings, trunk circles, bodyweight squats, or lunges. We will explore this further in the Mobility chapter.

After the workout, you should do static stretching, which we shall explore further in the flexibility chapter. I also recommend using a foam roller to perform a self-myofascial release massage either pre and/or post workout. This simply involves placing the roller between the muscle group you wish to work and the floor or a wall. You then roll back and forth to apply pressure to the muscle. The degree to which you push down on the roller dictates how deeply you penetrate the muscle tissue. We will also explore this further in the Mobility chapter.

Monday Workout – Upper Body

Pectorals, Latissimus Dorsi, Rhomboids, Trapezius, Deltoids, Rotator Cuff, Biceps, Triceps, Forearms

Exercise	Sets	Repetitions	Rest Between Sets
Decline Dumbbell Press	5	20/15/10/8/8	60-90 seconds
One Arm Lat Pull In	5	20/15/10/8/8	60-90 seconds
Shrugs	4	20/15/10/8	60-90 seconds
Rear Delt Cable Extension	4	20/15/10/8	60-90 seconds
Cable Deltoid Press	4	20/15/10/8	60-90 seconds
Decline Dumbbell Triceps Extension	4	20/15/10/8	60-90 seconds
Alternate Dumbbell Curl	4	20/16/10/8	60-90 seconds
Barbell Wrist Curl	3	20/15/10	60-90 seconds

Tuesday Workout – Lower Body and Core

Quadriceps, Glutes, Hamstrings, Calves, Abdominals, Obliques, Erector Spinae

Exercise	Sets	Repetitions	Rest Between Sets
Cable or Goblet Squat	5	20/15/10/8/8	60-90 seconds
Barbell Hip Thrusts or Glute kickback machine	5	20/15/10/8/8	60-90 seconds
Alternative Dumbbell Reverse Lunges	4	20,16,10,8	60-90 seconds
Seated Leg Curl	4	20/15/10/8	60-90 seconds
Seated or Standing Calf Raise	4	25/20/15/10	60-90 seconds
Cable Crunch	3	25/20/15	60-90 seconds
Cable Torso Rotation	3	15/15/15	60-90 seconds
Seated Torso Extension	3	25/20/15	60-90 seconds

SUMMARY

Strength training will form the main foundation of your total fitness program. Make it your goal to perfect your exercise form, really feeling the working muscles and concentrating on moving through a full range of motion. Challenge yourself to progressively increase the resistance you are working with so as to make consistent improvement in your strength and muscle mass. Do these things week in and week out, and you will be amazed at how much stronger, more muscular, energetic and vibrant you will look and feel.

Now it's time to discover how the next foundation will play its vital role in your health and fitness journey...

4

FLEXIBILITY - STRETCH TO IMPRESS

If you've ever marveled at the ability of children to put their feet behind their head or do the splits and then struggled to bend down to tie your shoes, you have become painfully aware of the effect that age has on flexibility. When we move into our 40s, we start to begin to notice that the things we used to take for granted are just that little bit more difficult to perform. These changes are subtle but there will come a point when you'll realize just how much flexibility you've lost.

The good news is that, while you may have lost some flexibility, it is not that difficult to find it again. Understanding what flexibility is, the different forms it takes, and when you should do each one is the key to reclaiming the flexibility of your youth.

WHAT IS FLEXIBILITY?

Flexibility is the ability of your joints to move freely through their complete range of motion. Flexibility training helps to improve the range of motion of your muscles.

If you don't have good flexibility, such everyday activities as getting out of bed, bending down to pick up a child or squatting down to lift a heavy or light object can become more demanding. A lack of adequate flexibility can also impair your athletic ability, as you will be unable to reach the full potential, strength and power of your muscles.

FLEXIBILITY BENEFITS

Increased Range of Motion: Range of motion is the distance and direction your joints can move. Consistent flexibility training will increase the range of motion of your joints and muscles. It does this by lengthening the muscles and opening the joints. As a result, you'll be able to stretch further in all directions while remaining pain free.

Decreased Risk of Injury: People with flexible muscles are less likely to become injured during physical activity.

Reduced Muscle Soreness: Flexibility training helps to reduce muscle soreness after you exercise. When you stretch after your workout, you keep your muscles loose and relaxed.

Improved Athletic Performance: When your joint and muscles are flexible, you use less energy in motion. This makes you more efficient, improving your performance.

WHY WE BECOME LESS FLEXIBLE WITH AGE

When most people enter their 40s, they notice a marked drop off in their flexibility. At the same time, their joints become achy. That's because, as we age, our ligaments are not as flexible as they used to be. The amount of synovial fluid inside the joints diminishes and the cartilage becomes thinner. This appears to be most prevalent around the hips and knees.

As we age, the tissue that surrounds our joints also thickens. This contributes to a lack of flexibility. The loss of muscle mass and the associated strength decline is another contributor to reduced flexibility as we age. In tandem with age related muscle loss, many people accumulate more stored body fat as they age, further exacerbating the lack of flexibility problem.

A simple thing we can all do to improve our flexibility is to drink more water. This will increase the lubrication of the joints, helping to offset the natural loss of synovial fluid that occurred with aging. Enhancing joint movement through exercise will also help to reverse cartilage shrinkage and increase mobility.

MOST COMMON FLEXIBILITY ISSUES FOR THE ELDERLY

Limited flexibility most commonly evidences itself in the elderly with reduced movement in the hips and spine. This is the cause of chronic and ongoing pain for millions of people. Though back pain can have a number of root causes, impaired flexibility in the hamstrings, glutes and hip flexors is often a major contributing factor.

When a person has tight hamstrings, these muscles will unnaturally pull the pelvis downward. This will result in lower back tension and soreness.

The hip flexor muscles are connected to the leg bones (femur or tibia) and the hip joint. They allow the knee to lift the thigh up and to the sides. The three main hip flexor muscles are the:

- Iliopsoas
- Sartorius
- Rectus Femoris

When we are in a sedentary, seated position for hours on end, our hips maintain a flexed position. The lack of movement of the hip flexors causes them cumulatively to shorten and shrink. Tightness in muscles such as the iliopsoas will cause you to compress your spine and tilt your pelvis forward - again leading to tension in the lower back.

The piriformis muscle is situated in the buttocks above the hip joint. It assists the hip flexors to lift and moves the thighs away from the body. Lack of flexibility can lead to piriformis syndrome, which is characterized by numbness and pain in the buttocks. As a result of the piriformis muscle pressing down on the sciatic nerve, many people also experience pain running down each leg, which is known as sciatica.

GENDER DIFFERENCES

Women naturally have greater hip flexibility than men do. This results from a greater preponderance of estrogenic hormones which are designed to prepare the female body for the rigors of childbirth. As a result, women have enhanced hip bone mobility through the pelvis, as well as better mobility through the tailbone. They also have a wider and more circular pelvis than men.

The bone and muscle changes that occur in females during puberty make their lower body joints less stable than male joints. One result of this is that, when resistance is applied to the quads and knees (such as when doing the squat), the knees tend to buckle inward.

Women also naturally have better shoulder joint mobility, especially through the anterior (front) deltoid's range of motion.

TYPES OF STRETCHING

Dynamic Stretching

It has become increasingly popular over recent years, as studies have shown the negative effects of static stretching on training performance before exercise. Dynamic stretching involves speed of movement, momentum and active muscular effort to perform a stretch. Often the stretch mimics or is closely linked to the upcoming athletic performance.

It is good to include some dynamic stretching in your warmup routine, regardless of the type of exercise you are doing, as it is a good way to reduce tightness in the muscles while upping the core temperature of the body and enhancing the range of motion around your joints. It also prepares your body for the specific demands of the activity that you will be performing during your training session. Examples of dynamic stretches include walking knee hugs, side lunges, ankle and wrist rotations, leg swings and torso twists. We shall explore this further in the next chapter.

Static Stretching

Static stretching, also known as isometric stretching, involves extending a muscle until you feel a gentle stretch. This is the best form of stretching to improve flexibility and is ideally done immediately after your strength training workout. You can also perform a separate static stretching session later in the day, taking more time to stretch for longer. If you are completing a separate stretching session, you should, as always, warm up your body for a few minutes before.

PNF Stretching

Proprioceptive Neuromuscular Facilitation (PNF) is an adaptation of static stretching. It involves both stretching and contracting the target muscle group. It is extremely effective at improving flexibility and increasing range of motion.

PNF stretching relies on the stretch reflex of the myotendinous unit by activating mechanoreceptors within the muscle called muscle spindle units and Golgi tendon organs. Muscle spindles help to regulate overall muscle length and tone by activating gamma motor neurons by way of the stretch reflex.

The initial isometric contraction (hold) phase of the PNF stretch lasts for 10 seconds at 40 percent maximal contraction. The muscle then relaxes into a passive stretch for 30 seconds. You repeat this 4 times then, on the 5th contraction, you hold the position for 15 seconds. With each repetition you slightly increase the stretch position.

Ballistic Stretching

Ballistic stretching involves stretching a muscle to where you feel a gentle stretch and then bouncing to extend the stretch even further. This form of stretching is NOT recommended as it carries a risk of injury to the muscle.

FLEXIBILITY TESTING

Before you begin a stretching program, you should determine your current level of flexibility. Retest every 8 weeks to gauge your progress.

Precede your tests with 5 minutes of light cardio exercise such as skipping or light running to ensure your muscles are warm.

Here are 4 examples:

Modified Sit & Reach Test

Lower Back and Hamstring Flexibility

For this test you will need a 30cm high box and a one meter rule.

Sit with your back against a wall and your legs outstretched and together. Have a friend position the box against your feet. Keeping your shoulder blades against the wall and your knees straight, stretch your arms forward. Have your friend put the meter rule on the box and move it forward until the end touches your fingertips. This is your zero point.

Now stretch forward as far as possible without bending your knees. Have your friend record the distance of your stretch on the meter rule. Do not bounce or jerk during the stretch.

Repeat the test three times and take the average.

Trunk Rotation Test

Trunk & Shoulder Flexibility

For this test you will need a wall and a piece of chalk.

Stand in front of a wall and mark a vertical line on it. Stand facing away from the wall in front of the line, arm's length away from it. Extend your arms in front of your torso. Now twist your torso to the left and touch the wall behind you with your fingertips. Mark this point with the chalk. Measure the distance from the line. A point before the line is a negative score and a point after the line is a positive score.

Repeat on the right side and then take the average of the two scores.

Groin Flexibility Test

Groin Flexibility

You will need a ruler for this test.

Sit on the floor with knees bent, and your legs together with feet flat on the floor. Keeping your feet together, drop your knees down to the sides. Now grab your feet with both hands and pull your ankles toward your body. Have a friend measure the distance between your heels and your groin.

Thomas Test

Hip Flexibility

You will need a ruler for this test.

Lie supine (on your back) on a table with both lower legs hanging off the end (knees flexed). Bring your right knee towards your chest and hold just below the knee with both hands. Keep your lower back flat on the table if you can. If there is no tightness in the left hip, the leg will remain flat on the table. If there is tightness, then the left leg will rise off the table. Ask a friend to use the ruler to measure how high your left leg is off the table. Repeat on the other leg. Here are 4 things to look out for:

- Increased lumbar lordosis (arch of the lower back) could mean tight hip flexors.
- If you are unable to bring the hip into full extension so it rests in the air could mean tight hip flexors.
- If you are unable to bring the knee to 90 degree flexion and hold it in place could mean tight quadriceps.
- If your knee drifts to the side into hip abduction, this could also mean a tight TFL muscle.

STRETCHING RECOMMENDATIONS

- The American College of Sports Medicine (ACSM) recommends flexibility exercises for all of the major muscle-tendon groups - neck, shoulders, trunk, lower back, hips, legs, ankles - 2-3 times per week.
- Spend up to 60 seconds on each stretch; if you can only hold the stretch for 20 seconds, repeat the stretch three times.
- Never bounce into a stretch.
- Perform dynamic stretches before your workout.
- Perform static stretching after your workout.
- If you are doing a separate stretching session, do a 5 minute warm up of cardio and dynamic stretches.

16 GREAT STATIC STRETCHES

N.B. Always stretch both sides for the same amount of time!

Neck Stretch

Bend your head forward so that your chin touches your upper chest. Bend your head backwards so that you are looking at the ceiling. Bend your head to the left side, trying to get your ear to touch your shoulder. Repeat this on the right side. Hold for 60 seconds each.

Latissimus Dorsi Stretch

Place both hands face down on a fence, ledge or mantel. Bending at the waist, let your body drop down while keeping your knees slightly bent and arms straight out in front of you. Hold this gentle stretch for 60 seconds.

Spinal Stretch

Start by kneeling on your hands and knees. Push your hips back, so your pelvis sinks between your knees and your head rests on the floor. Extend your hands out as far as you can in front of you. Hold for 60 seconds.

Oblique Stretch

Standing - Lean to the right, keeping your left arm straight over your head, and right arm on your hip. Hold for 60 seconds.

Arms, Shoulders & Chest Stretch

Grab a towel at both ends while keeping your arms straight. Without bending your arms, raise the towel over your head and behind your back. Hold the towel behind your back for 60 seconds.

Pectoral Stretch

Standing – Place your right forearm onto a door frame so that your fingertips are pointing toward the ceiling. Your upper arm should be at shoulder height with your elbow bent at 90 degrees. Place your right foot forward and rotate your torso away from the frame. Hold for 60 seconds and repeat with the left arm.

Forearm & Wrist Stretch

Get down on your hands and knees. Turn your hands outwards until your thumbs are on the outside and your fingers are pointed towards your knees. Keeping your arms straight, start to lean backwards until you feel an easy stretch in your forearms. Hold for 60 seconds.

Hip Flexor Stretch

Start by kneeling on a mat, then place your right foot forward so that you have a 90-degree angle at the hip and knee. The left knee should remain on the floor, aligned underneath the left hip. Place your hands on the right knee for support (if needed). Keeping the torso upright, slightly tuck your pelvis under. Slowly lean forward until you feel a comfortable stretch in front of your left hip. Hold for 60 seconds.

Quad Stretch

Standing - Hold your foot at the lace part of your shoe (not your ankle), bring it behind your body and tuck your pelvis under so your tailbone is pointing at the wall in front of you (a posterior tilt). Try and get your heel to touch your glute without letting your knee swing out to the side. Hold for 60 seconds.

Hamstring Stretch

Standing - With your feet hip width apart, place your right leg forward so your right heel is just in front of your left toe. Keeping your right leg straight, place your hands on your left knee and bend the knee. With a straight back, gently lean forward resting your weight on your bent leg. Hold for 60 seconds.

Glute Stretch

Sit on a chair and cross your right ankle just above your left knee. Place your hands on the inner side of your right knee, lean forward slightly and apply gentle pressure. Hold for 60 seconds.

Groin Stretch

Sit on the floor with the soles of your feet together while grabbing them with your hands. Your heels should be a comfortable distance (for you) from your crotch. Gently pull yourself forward, keeping your back straight, until you feel an easy stretch in your groin. Hold for 60 seconds.

Abductor Stretch

Standing - lean forward and grab onto a chair for balance. Cross one foot behind the other and slide that foot away from your body, keeping your legs straight. Slowly bend your front leg to lower your body. Hold for 60 seconds.

Calf Stretch I

Position the ball of your foot on the edge of a stair. Your other foot should be completely on the stair and you may wish to grab a railing or wall for balance. Lower the heel of your foot below the stair level. Hold for 60 seconds.

Calf Stretch II

Stand facing a wall and place your palms on it in line with your chest. Step your right leg back so that it is fully extended with your left knee slightly bent. Now lean forward to the wall, keeping your back foot completely on the floor. You should feel the stretch through your calf muscle. Hold for 60 seconds.

The World's Greatest Stretch

This stretch does indeed live up to its moniker, as it stretches almost every major muscle group in some way. It has been modified over the years and you can find numerous variations online. Here is a relatively easy version to follow:

1. Standing hip width apart, lunge forward with your right leg and put your left hand on the ground opposite the right leg. You will now be in a balanced half kneeling or exaggerated sprint position. Your front (right) knee should be directly above your ankle and back (left) ankle behind your toe.

2. Keeping your left leg as straight as you can, lower your right forearm to the ground and hold for 10 seconds.
3. Keeping your hips still and in line with your back (left) leg, extend your right arm up to 90 degrees towards the ceiling, rotating your torso. Look up and hold for 10 seconds. Try to keep your back foot still as you rotate.
4. Bring your right arm down and rotate underneath your torso to the left. Hold for 10 seconds.

Repeat this action 10 times and switch sides.

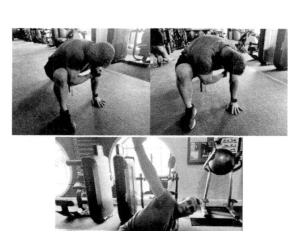

YOGA FOR FLEXIBILITY

Yoga is an all-encompassing term which describes a system of wellbeing that originated in ancient India. Yoga embraces breathing exercises, relaxation and meditation techniques and physical movement. In terms of flexibility improvement, it is *hatha*, or physical yoga that is our focus.

Yoga is a smart choice for people wanting to improve their flexibility. It provides a gentle journey through your comfort zone, without forcing your body. Being a low impact form of exercise, yoga is accessible to all people, be they seasoned athletes or couch potatoes.

Yoga provides a holistic approach to stretching. Conventional stretching stretches one muscle group at a time. However, hatha yoga unites the person, synchronizing the body, the breath and the mind.

Yoga will make you more flexible, which will, in turn, make you more agile. And, a more agile body is a more balanced, stronger body. Agility refers to the body's ability to change direction and position of the body fluidly without physical or mental strain. The bending, rotating and pivoting involved in yoga will keep you agile all day long.

Your body balance and proprioception, which relates to your awareness of your body's position in space, are also heightened by yoga training.

Yoga Positioning

Body positioning is integral to successful yoga practice. There are three parts to every yoga pose:

1. Movement into the pose
2. Stillness while holding the pose
3. Movement out of the pose

Each of these areas are equally important. Unless your positioning is on point, you are likely to cause injury to your muscles and joints.

As a beginner, you need to perfect your yoga positioning. How can you do it?

I suggest joining a yoga studio for a month in order to learn the proper technique.

SUMMARY

We have now discovered the issues that are inherent with a lack of flexibility as we age, but more importantly, the benefits of exercise and strategies as simple as hydration for improving our flexibility. You can perform dynamic stretches at the beginning of a workout to help your muscles warm up; static stretches at the end of a gym session, which will help your muscles recover from exercise; and also longer stretching sessions on their own at home when you are watching TV, or listening to music or audiobooks. The key is to make sure that however you do it, you are stretching regularly and gently. Flexibility does take time to achieve and requires a lot of patience, but you will get there with time! The key, as with all my 7 foundations, is consistency. In our next chapter we will explore another key foundation of total fitness that flexibility is essential to help maintain. Luckily for us, this next foundation is more dynamic, and in my opinion can be a lot of fun to train.

Let's get moving...

5

MOBILITY - MOVE IT OR LOSE IT!

Loss of mobility is one of the classic signs of aging. In fact, it's a stereotype of people over the age of 60. They are expected to be mobility challenged, to stumble and fall at the slightest obstacle. Yet, as we discovered earlier, loss of mobility is not an inevitable sign of aging. Mobility, the ability to move your body freely through a range of motion without pain, can be maintained and even enhanced by maintaining daily exercise habits, controlling your weight and following a balanced diet.

THE IMPORTANCE OF MOBILITY

A mobile person is able to maintain control over the contraction of their muscles throughout the whole of a joint movement. For instance, when you straighten out your elbow and then bend it so that your fist comes up to your shoulder, you are flexing and extending the elbow joint by contracting the biceps muscles. If you are mobile, your muscles will be strong and flexible enough to move the joint through its whole range of motion in a controlled manner, as well as to stop and hold the movement at any given point. Essentially, being mobile means that you have total control over your joints and muscles.

When you establish a base of mobility, you are able to build strength and explosiveness and realize your potential in any exercise or sporting pursuit that you put your mind to. In fact, mobility underpins all of the benefits of strength training that were detailed in the previous chapter. If you are lacking in mobility, you will struggle to perform the strength training exercises that were laid out in that chapter. It makes sense, then, to follow a mobility enhancement routine in tandem with your strength training.

Lack of mobility is a major contributor to falls in the elderly. Combine this with loss of muscular strength, stability and flexibility and it's not hard to understand why falls have become the leading cause of traumatic death over the age of 65 in the United States. Yet, the combination of mobility and strength training will dramatically offset the lack of mobility and subsequent balance problems that many people think are part and parcel of getting older.

People who are able to maintain a high level of mobility as they move into their 60s and 70s experience a much greater sense of freedom, independence and overall quality of life. In contrast, those who suffer from limited mobility experience pain every time they move a muscle and have to put up with creaky joints. They can't help but feel that their zest for life and energy is slowly but consistently being drained away.

Importantly, elderly people who have a good level of mobility are able to live independently for longer. They are able to carry out their everyday tasks without assistance, cook for themselves, play with their grandkids, and enjoy leisure activities outside of the home. This has a huge psychological benefit, allowing them to stay connected, feel part of things and really enjoy their golden years and everything that they have to offer.

Why We Become Less Mobile As We Age

Loss of mobility as we age is a combination of the following factors:

- Age related muscle loss ('sarcopenia')
- Loss of bone mass
- Reduction in range of joint motion
- Accumulation of body fat
- Lack of physical movement
- Poor dietary habits

As we think about each of these factors, we realize that they can all be offset through our lifestyle habits. Sure, the first three factors are a natural part of aging. We will all lose between 3-8 percent of our muscle mass every decade after the age of 30; by the age of 40, each of us will begin to lose joint movement - our hip joint flexion will decrease by 6-7 degrees per decade, and concurrently our shoulder range of motion will go down by 5-6 degrees. Yet, the right type of strength and mobility exercises can help to offset those natural losses. There are many thousands of examples of men and women in their 40s, 50s and 60s who are stronger, have more muscle AND greater mobility than they did in their 20s and 30s.

Obesity is a major risk factor for the loss of mobility. An obese person puts far greater demands on his skeletal muscles than a healthy weight person does. High levels of adipose tissue (fat) have also been associated with reduced functional muscle ability and strength. Lack of flexibility and control over muscles is also more readily seen among overweight individuals.

TYPICAL MOBILITY ISSUES

Mobility problems usually manifest themselves as difficulty with walking or maintaining a healthy posture. Balance issues are also common with people as they age. In fact, this is the number one reason that elderly people make appointments to see their doctor. Not all balance issues, however, are mobility related. Vertigo, inner ear problems and nerve conditions may also be at the root of the problem.

Postural problems that are linked to lack of mobility typically exacerbate with age. When you are standing with a normal posture your spine will have a normal forward curvature. This is called 'kyphosis'. This is matched by reverse curvature ('lordosis') in the cervical and lumbar spine. These natural curvatures allow us to sit up and stand with ideal positioning.

Postural problems occur when we develop an exaggerated forward curvature of the upper spine. This has become a huge problem in recent decades as a result of our computer dominant lifestyles. Most people spend more than an hour each day hunched over some form of technology nowadays. The excessive forward curvature that develops as a result is known as 'hyperkyphosis'.

Something as simple as doing daily scapular retractions can be a huge help! You can do these by sitting or standing upright and squeezing your shoulder blades down and back so they move closer together. This will also make your chest look bigger which is an extra bonus! Just be careful not to lean back as it will hyperextend your lumbar spine (lower back). You can modify this by extending your elbows and fingers to create a mountain pose. This is the complete opposite of what we do in our day to day lives as you are focusing on thoracic extension rather than flexion.

IMPROVING YOUR MOBILITY

Improving your mobility should be something that fits seamlessly into your exercise program. In other words, it doesn't have to be a separate workout in its own right (though it can be) but, rather, can be included as an extension of your strength training workout. Mobility training should include the following elements:

- Myofascial tissue massage to release and loosen muscles
- Dynamic stretching
- Mobility drills

Perform your mobility work as part of your warm-up to your strength training session. The total duration of your mobility warm-up should ideally be around 10 minutes.

SELF MYOFASCIAL RELEASE

Self-Myofascial Release (SMR) is a form of self-massage which has become hugely popular among runners and exercise enthusiasts due to its ease of application and immediacy of result. SMR involves alleviating soft-tissue stiffness and pain hot spots with a form of self-massage. It has also proven to be a great post-workout recovery aid.

SMR makes use of a simple massage aid, such as a foam roller or massage ball, to manipulate and put pressure on muscle sore spots. In addition to its rehabilitative ability SMR has been shown to improve flexibility and exercise performance.

To understand how SMR manages to achieve its quite remarkable outcomes with such a seemingly simple procedure, we need to delve into the mysteries of the body's kinetic chain. The kinetic chain refers to the interconnected soft tissue, neural and articular systems. If any one of these systems is not working optimally, the other systems compensate by working harder. If left unchecked, this will lead to tissue overload, fatigue, pain and restricted mobility.

SMR works on the two neural receptors that are found in your muscles, the muscle spindle and the golgi tendon organ. Muscle spindles, located parallel to muscle fibers, send messages to the central nervous system about fiber length changes as a result of injury, which triggers the myotatic stretch reflex. The result? Pain.

Golgi tendon organ overstimulation can likewise lead to inhibited movement and soreness. Soft tissue massage focused on these receptors provides immediate relief from pain, restores normal fiber length and improves function.

Using a Foam Roller

A foam roller is a cylindrical piece of high density foam. The most basic form is a flat edged EPE soft roller. Trigger Point Grid Foam rollers are firmer and feature grooves, indentations and protrusions that allow you to penetrate your trigger points.

Find an open space that allows freedom of movement. Place the roller on the floor and position your body so that the area of focus is on top of the roller. The pressure that massages the affected area will be provided by your body.

Gently roll your body back and forth over the roller. Your focus should be on areas of tightness and those that have a reduced range of motion - if you feel a tight spot, hold the stretch there for a few seconds. Control this pressure by adjusting the amount of bodyweight that you place on the roller. You can use your hands and feet to offset the weight as needed.

Here are most effective foam rolling moves for your major muscle groups:

Quadriceps

Rest one leg on the ground and place the other thigh over the edge of the foam roller, just above the knee. Support your body on your palms and elbows. Now roll the thigh up and down by pushing your hips back. As you roll, place pressure on all four of the quadriceps muscles to emphasize that area.

Hamstrings

Sit on the floor with the foam roller resting under one hamstring just above the knee. Support your body by resting your palms on the floor behind you. Now move up and down the roller from your knees to your hips by pushing your hips back and forth.

Calves

Sit on the floor with the foam roller resting under one calf just below the knee. Support your body by resting your palms on the floor behind you. Now move up and down the roller from your knee to your ankle by pushing your hips back and forth.

IT Band/TFL

Lie on the floor sideways with one hip resting on the foam roller. Bend your other knee with the sole of your foot on the floor. Start rolling from the bottom of the thigh, just above your knee, and come up to the outer part of the hip.

Back

Lie on the floor with the foam roller under your shoulder blades. Roll up and down your back with slow, smooth movements. Try to avoid going any lower than your ribs as the lower back is a more vulnerable area. If you have a specific trigger point area in your back, you may want to use a tennis ball to apply direct pressure to that area. You can also do this standing against a wall. This is particularly useful for the lower back as you are able to better control the pressure.

Chest

Lie face down on the foam roller, with it directly underneath your sternum (breastplate) and orientated so it points towards your head. With your arm out to the side, you can then roller down the length of the pectoral muscles from the sternum to your armpit. This stretch is most useful for men - if you are a woman and you find this impractical, you can use a tennis ball against a wall and apply pressure point massage as needed.

DYNAMIC STRETCHING

Dynamic stretching involves moving your muscles through their full range of motion. Dynamic stretches often simulate the resistance moves that are part of the workout to come, such as doing bodyweight squats or lunges.

Here is a 5 move dynamic stretching routine that will enhance your mobility ahead of your workout:

Bodyweight Squats w/high knees x 10

Stand with your feet shoulder width apart and your arms extended out in front of you. Maintain a neutral spine, then hinge from the hips to lower down into a parallel squat position. Push through the heels to return to the start position. You can also add in alternate high knees or mini kicks as a good modification.

Overhead Twisting Reverse Lunge x 5 (each side)

From the same starting position, take a large step backwards with your left leg and lower down into a lunge position. Now, keeping your arms straight overhead, twist your torso to the right then back to the center. Push back through the right thigh to return to the start position. After 5 reps, repeat on the right leg.

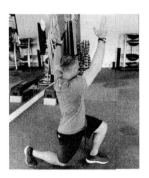

Superman x 10

Lie face down on an exercise mat with your body in an arched position so that your arms and feet are extended off the ground in a dish shape. Now arch up to full extension to bring your arms and feet up as high as possible. Lower and repeat.

Arm Circles x 20

Stand with your arms hanging at your sides. Now rotate from the shoulder joint to move your arms in wide circles at the sides of your body. Keep the elbows locked and concentrate on achieving a 360 degree range of motion.

World's Greatest Stretch – Dynamic x 10

As mentioned earlier in the flexibility chapter, The World's Greatest Stretch is one of the best all round stretches you can do. However this can also be done as a dynamic stretch by simply performing the steps outlined in chapter 4 but without holding the positions and alternating legs after each movement pattern. Two extra points to consider are

1. Try not to raise your hips when you switch legs.
2. Keep the flow of the movements smooth and focus on regulating your breathing.

MOBILITY DRILLS

Perform your mobility drills immediately after your dynamic stretching exercises. Perform 10 reps on each movement and then go straight into the next exercise. Once you've finished these, you'll be ready to get cracking with your training session!

Cat cows

Start on your hands and knees. Your knees directly under your hips and hands under your shoulders and with your spine neutral. As you inhale, move into cow pose by sticking your bum out and pressing your chest forward and allowing your upper back to sink. Lift your head looking forward and relax your shoulders away from your ears. Now exhale into cat pose by rounding your spine towards the ceiling and tucking in your tailbone. Relax your head and lower toward your chin. Repeat 10 times.

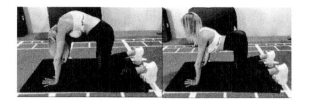

Walkouts

Stand with your feet hip to shoulder width apart and with good posture. Start to reach down to the ground with your hands and only bend your knees when you need to. This will give you a nice stretch in your hamstrings. Walk your hands out in front of you and keep your knees in line with your toes. Do this until you are in a perfect press up plank position. Hold for 2 seconds. Walk your hands back up towards your body to reverse the movement.

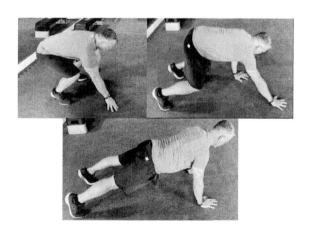

Standing hip circles

Standing tall, place your hands on your hips and feet slightly apart. Start to make a clockwise circular motion with your hips from left to right. Repeat 10 times then change direction.

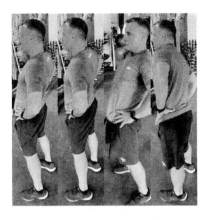

Leg swings

Stand sideways next to a wall, chair, door handle so you have plenty of room. Hold on with your hand next to the support and your outside hand on your hip. Keep your back upright and core engaged. Start to swing your furthest leg forward and back like a pendulum. Start slowly at first with a small range of motion and start to increase the range as the reps go up. You ideally want to get to a full range of motion at the hip but not so high that your back bends and your hip starts to rotate. 15 - 20 swings on each leg.

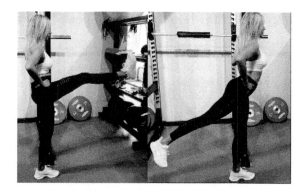

Lying Can openers

Lie on your right side and bend both knees. You can use a foam block in between the knees to help hip alignment and for your head to keep your neck neutral. Have both arms in front of your body with both hands touching. Keep your shoulder blades relaxed. Take your top (right) arm and rotate it round to the left till your back is as flat as possible. This action will rotate your torso. Try not to let your knees come off the ground or away from each other. Repeat 10 times then switch sides.

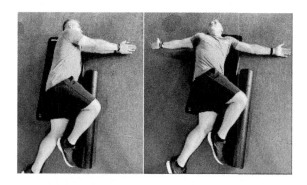

Dynamic crucifix

Lie down on a mat with straight legs and extend your arms out to the side so they are in line with your shoulders. Lift your right leg off the ground and bend your knee. Rotate it across your body to the left. Ideally your right hip should be facing the ceiling. Touch the floor with your right foot keeping your back as flat as you can. Switch directions and alternate 10 times.

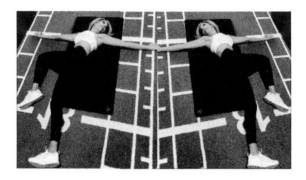

Fire hydrants

Start on your hands and knees. Your knees directly under your hips and hands under your shoulders and with your spine neutral and engaged. Keeping your torso and left leg completely still. Lift your right knee and raise it sideways away from your body. Bring it back to the starting position. Repeat 12 – 15 times.

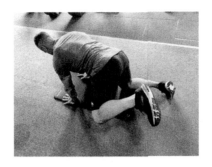

SUMMARY

Improving your mobility will do wonders for your enjoyment of life and your everyday functionality. Whether it's gardening, DIY or playing with your kids in the back yard. Getting there is not that difficult. In fact, the three-part routine (foam rolling, dynamic stretching and mobility drills) that we've covered in this chapter takes just a few minutes to complete. Add it in as part of your warm up before your strength training and you will be amazed at how much more fluid, mobile and free you will feel - try it and see for yourself! You can also perform these three aspects as a separate routine to wake you up in the morning. Your heart rate will increase while you do this, so it's a great jump start to the day.

In the next chapter, you will discover the benefits of yet another foundation and why its relationship with mobility is so important...

6

STABILITY - FINDING THE BALANCE

Falls are the number one cause of injury in people aged 60 and over. They can result in everything from pelvic fractures to head injuries, or even death. Scarily, 25% of people in this age bracket experience at least one fall per year.

But why do we fall?

Some falls are due to environmental factors (e.g. poor lighting, inappropriate footwear, or uneven surfaces), but the major issue for most people is one simple factor: a lack of stability. Stability describes our ability to control our body during movement. You can consider stability as the framework of a car. When you improve your body's stability system, you are developing a strong foundation to support your body's engine.

THE STABILITY-MOBILITY CONTINUUM

The joints of our body can move in three different planes of motion - the sagittal plane (flexion and extension, i.e. bending and straightening), the frontal plane (abduction and adduction, i.e. moving towards and away from the centerline of the body) and the transverse plane (rotation). Some joints are more mobile than others, moving in all three planes of motion (for example, our shoulders and hips). In comparison, joints like the knees and elbows are very stable, moving only in the sagittal plane. Your body needs a combination of mobile and stable joints in order to function effectively. In fact, the body alternates stable and mobile regions, which we can see if we look at the body as a chain from the ground up:

> Ankle (mobile) > knee (stable) > hip (mobile) > lumbar region (stable) > thoracic region (mobile) > scapulothoracic joint (stable) > shoulder (mobile) > elbow (stable) > wrist (mobile)

In a normal situation, these stable and mobile regions work in tandem; however, if there is a change in any one of these regions, this has a knock-on effect on the rest of the chain and can result in an injury that is seemingly unrelated to the affected area! If a normally mobile joint has sub-optimal mobility, one of the more stable joints nearby will need to work to compensate to provide the missing movement.

For example, if your ankle lacks mobility, often the knee will compensate, resulting in knee pain. Similarly, if you lose mobility in your hips or thoracic region, this can lead to low back pain because the normally stable lumbar spine needs to provide additional movement so you can perform your everyday functions.

But it's not quite as black and white as pure 'mobile' and 'stable' regions. Every joint, no matter how mobile, needs some stability. And the opposite is also true - even very stable joints like the lumbar spine need to have some mobility! We should therefore consider every joint as located somewhere on a stability-mobility continuum.

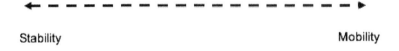

Stability   Mobility

Each joint needs a specific balance of stability and mobility - even joints such as the shoulder and ankle that require large amounts of mobility need some stability to prevent pain and injury. In reality, our joints are placed on the stability-mobility continuum as shown below:

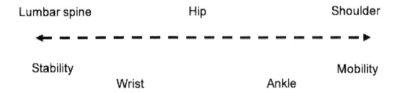

Ligament damage (such as a strain) can decrease the passive stability of a joint by making the ligaments more lax - this will improve mobility, but at the expense of necessary structural stability of the joint. This will put the joint at risk of further injury, and is one of the reasons that previous injury is one of the biggest predictors of future injury risk. It's also why it is so important for us to incorporate stability work into our exercise programming for total fitness.

KEEPING OUR BODY STABLE

There are three systems that help us keep our body stable: the proprioceptive, the visual, and the vestibular.

1. The Proprioceptive System. This system provides you with an awareness of where your body is in space and how much strength you need to perform a movement (for example, you need less force to open a crisp packet than to lift your grandchild into their car seat). This sense of perception and awareness of your body's position is crucial for you to engage effectively with your environment, as the information transmitted from sensory receptors to the brain dictates our muscle movement and actions.
2. The Visual System. We use our vision to detect information about our surroundings - for example, our location, direction, speed of

movement, obstacles, and the surface we are moving on.
3. The Vestibular System. This system is located within our inner ear, and consists of three fluid-filled channels. Movement of the neck causes movement of the fluid in these channels, which helps our brain detect our body position. It also allows us to determine the position and location of objects surrounding us.

As we age, the function of all of these systems becomes less efficient, leading to a gradual loss of stability with time. Reductions in the capacity of the visual and vestibular system come with the loss of vision and hearing often experienced with age, and they can also be a side-effect of disease or neurological conditions. The proprioceptive system also experiences declines, which impacts our movement as a whole - you are likely to walk slower, for example, if your body isn't sure where your foot is in relation to the ground. Together with the loss of muscle size and strength with age (known as sarcopenia), this drastically increases our risk of falling as we grow older.

Luckily for us, we now know that we can slow down this loss of muscle size and strength using resistance training. However, while strength training is key, it's not enough on its own. Unfortunately, there may not be much we can do to change the visual or vestibular systems, but we can supplement our training with exercises designed specifically to target the proprioceptive system. This will improve our stability through movement, reducing our risk of joint injuries, and as we get older, falls.

IMPROVING YOUR STABILITY

Now we know why stability is so important for reducing the risk of joint injuries and falls, we should consider how we can program exercise to improve our stability. There are two aspects of stability that need to be trained:

- Active Stability
- Passive Stability

Active stability relates to the body's mechanism for movement based on the signals that are sent from the brain. When you improve your active stability, you enhance your strength, mobility and stamina. We can improve our active stability by performing balance exercises.

Passive stability relates to the actual movement of your cartilage, bones and ligaments. We can consider these components to be the hardware of movement. Improving your passive stability through strength training will allow you to perform movement more fluidly.

Thinking about the regions that we described above as needing stability (i.e. knee, lower back, scapulothoracic region and elbow), we can see that the most important muscles you need to train to improve your body's stability are...

Lower Body

- The Core (abdominals and lumbar spine)
- The Quadriceps
- The Glutes

Upper Body

- Rotator cuff

Below are some simple exercises designed to target these muscle groups and train your joint stability. All you will need is an exercise band.

LOWER BODY

3 Types of Bridges - Targeting Hip Stability

1. Two Leg Bridge

Lie on your back with both knees bent and your feet flat on the floor hip width apart. Perform a slight tuck of your pelvis, making your lower back flat and depressing your lower ribs (imagine squashing a grape with your lower back). Focus on holding this posture. Squeeze your glutes to lift your hips up whilst also pressing down with your heels. Stop when you feel like you are unable to control your hips (i.e. if you start wobbling). The height is not important with this exercise, so do not try to go too high. When you can lift your hips up to form a straight line with the rest of your torso in a well-controlled manner. Make sure that your knees stay as wide as your feet. Hold the top position for two to three seconds and repeat 12 times.

2. Marching Bridge with Band

Perform the same two-legged bridge as in the last exercise but pause with your hips in the elevated position. Perform slow alternating kick ups by straightening your leg, as though you were marching. Use a light resistance band around your knees and focus on maintaining the tension on the band throughout the exercise. Make sure your knees stay still and your hips stay level! 20 Repetitions in total

3. One Leg Bridge

To perform a one leg bridge, lie on your back, feet hip width apart with one leg elevated with a 90 degree bend to your hip and knee. The leg will maintain this position during the movement. Perform your bridge pattern but on the single leg. Make sure your hips remain level left to right. Try 10 repetitions on each leg.

One Leg Balance - Targeting Lower Limb (Hip, Knee, Ankle)

Stand with your feet shoulder width apart. Now lift your left foot one inch from the floor. Maintain a straight spinal position as you hold for 15 seconds. Your goal should be to maintain an upright position without leaning to either side. Do 5 repetitions on each foot. You can make this more challenging by balancing on an unstable surface like dense foam or a BOSU ball and by raising your knee to hip height.

Hip Marching - Targeting Hips

Sit on a chair with your feet flat on the floor. Now lift your left knee as high as you can. Lower and repeat on the other leg. Perform 10 repetitions on each leg. To make this exercise slightly harder, resist your upward lift with your hands.

Lunges - Targeting Lower Limb (Hip, Knee, Ankle)

Stand with your feet hip width apart and your hands on your hips. Take a large step forward with your right leg, being sure to maintain an upright torso position but do not lean back. Lower your rear knee down as far as comfortable without it touching the floor. Now push back through the forward thigh to return to your standing start position. Perform 10 repetitions on each leg.

Airplanes - Targeting Core and Lower Limb (Hip, Knee, Ankle)

From a standing position, balance on one leg. Hinge your hips back with the other leg moving behind you. Keep the back leg in line with your torso as it lowers. Place your arms out to the side to balance your body, like wings on a plane. Keep a neutral spine. Hold this position for a few seconds, go back to the starting position and repeat. To make it more challenging try and stay on one leg during the whole set. You can also add a high knee in at the starting position as another modification. This can be a very challenging exercise to start with so by all means hold on to a chair with one arm at first if you need to until you feel more confident. Try 5 repetitions each side at first.

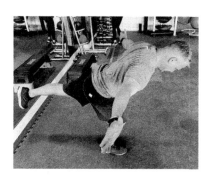

UPPER BODY

Scapulothoracic stability is incredibly important. The scapular stabilizer muscles control your shoulder blades. By coordinating with the rotator cuff (the muscles around your shoulder joint) they control how your arm moves. There are 17 muscles that work around the scapulothoracic joint. Five of the major muscles are:

- The Rhomboids
- Serratus Anterior
- Trapezius
- Levator Scapulae
- Latissimus Dorsi

Weakness in any of these major muscles will affect your shoulder function and how your scapula moves.

As always, there is good news. Here are some great exercises to help aid scapulothoracic stability:

ITYWs

Lie on your tummy face down on the floor keeping your arms to your sides. Make sure your neck is straight. Keep your body still: do not move anything other than your arms and follow these 4 steps by using the letters of the alphabet. *Hold all 4 positions for 10- 15 seconds each or do them dynamically in reps of 10 each.*

1. **I:** Hands down by your sides to create a letter "I", keep palms up and thumbs towards your thighs. Hold position or move them up and down (if doing reps).
2. **T:** Hold your hands out to the sides to create the letter "T" with your arms and body. Hold position or move your arms up and down (if doing reps) with your palms facing ground.
3. **Y:** Now move your arms up in a "Y" position. Hold position or move them up and down (if doing reps) with your palms down.
4. **W:** From the "Y" position, pull your arms into your body leading with the elbows finishing at sides to create a "W." Hold position or move your elbows up and down (if doing reps) squeezing

your shoulder blades as you pull down into your body. Repeat sequence 3 times.

Shoulder Blade Squeezes (Scapular Retraction)

Start by relaxing your neck. Stand with feet shoulder width apart and with good posture. Now slowly squeeze your shoulders back and slightly down to avoid shrugging your shoulders. Keep your abdominals and glutes braced. *Hold for 10 - 15 sec before relaxing your shoulders. Repeat 10 -12 times.*

Band Pull Apart

Stand tall with feet shoulder width apart. Holding a long resistance band with both hands with your palms facing each other and shoulder-width apart. Make sure there is no tension in the band yet. Pull the band apart with both arms to sides as wide as possible, keeping them just below shoulder height squeeze your shoulder blades together and down. Imagine you are trying to stop a tennis ball rolling down your back with your shoulder blades. With tension and control bring your hands back together to starting position. Repeat 12- 15 times.

ADDING STABILITY INTO GYM ROUTINES

As well as these more home based stability exercises, you can also challenge your body by tweaking your everyday resistance exercises at the gym. These could be, weighted single arm and leg exercises or using a Physio (Swiss) or Bosu ball. Here are some examples...

Swiss or Medicine Wall Ball Circles

With your feet shoulder width apart, face a wall holding a Swiss or medicine ball with one arm. Keep the ball shoulder height and press into the wall. Start to roll the ball clockwise making 10 circles. Do the same anti-clockwise and repeat 3 times.

Dumbbell Back Lunges with High Knee

Stand with your feet hip width apart, holding a dumbbell in each hand. Step back into a lunge with your right leg keeping your thigh at the same angle as your torso. Lower your right knee as low as you can go without hitting the ground. Now push back toward the starting position through the left thigh and raising your right knee. Your right knee is now parallel with your hip whilst balancing on your left leg. Hold for 2 seconds, repeat on the same leg for 10 repetitions, then swap legs.

Single Arm Lateral Raise

Stand with your feet hip width apart holding a dumbbell in one hand by your side. Raise your arm out to the side until it's parallel with your shoulder. Hold for 3 seconds. Lower your arm back down for 3 seconds keeping your torso completely still. Repeat 10 times and swap arms.

Single Arm Dumbbell Chest Press

Grab a single dumbbell and lie down on a gym bench. Extend your arm above you so that the dumbbell is over your shoulders but do not lock your elbow joint. Place your other hand on your hip. Slowly bring the dumbbell down to the side of your chest keeping your elbow slightly tucked. Keep your torso still. At the bottom position your elbow should form a right angle to your upper arms. Push back up to bring the dumbbell back to the starting position. Repeat 10 times then swap arms.

Dumbbell Chest Press on a Swiss/ physio ball

Grab a pair of dumbbells and lie down with your upper back on the ball, knees bent with your feet on the ground. Extend your arms above you so that the dumbbells are over your shoulders but do not lock your elbow joints. Slowly bring the dumbbells down to the side of your lower chest. In the bottom position your elbows should form a right angle to your upper arms. Push back up to bring the dumbbells together in the top position. Repeat 12 times.

Squats on a Bosu Ball

Place the blue side of the BOSU ball on the floor. Slowly step onto the flat side, standing with your feet wider than hip-width apart. Slowly push your hips back and bend your knees as you lower down into a squat. Hold for 3 seconds at the bottom. Push through your heels to stand back up to the starting position. Repeat 12 times.

Step Ups with High Knee (alternate legs)

Set up a step to a height that you are able to step onto comfortably. Place one foot on the step and push through your heel to lift your back leg off the ground. Follow through with your back leg raising your knee so it's parallel with your hip and standing tall on the other leg. Step back down and repeat with the other leg. Hold a dumbbell in each hand as a progression. 20 alternating repetitions.

Pallof Press

Fasten a resistance band to a secure anchor point in your gym or at home. Hold the end of the resistance band firmly in both hands. Position yourself away from the anchor point, with the resistance band held at chest height. Keep your feet shoulder-width apart, your knees slightly bent. Keep your feet firmly pushing down into the floor (scrunching your toes helps).Press the resistance band away from your chest, fully extending your arms in front of you without locking your elbows. Hold the resistance band at full extension for 2 - 3 seconds, and slowly release the tension. Return the band to the starting point, and repeat the exercise 12 times. You can also do this as a single arm exercise.

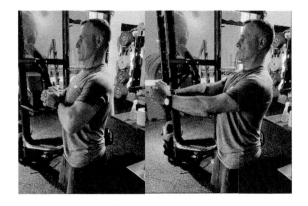

SUMMARY

Improving your stability is perhaps the most important thing you can do to reduce the likelihood that you will become another fall victim. And the great news is, doing so doesn't require a lot of effort. Performing some of these home exercises a couple of times a week can make a huge difference. It can also just take a few minutes - in fact, you can even do them during the ads on TV, or as a quick morning/ before bed routine. Adding the more gym-based exercises into your routine will also play a huge role in your increased stability and strength.

This is all another piece of the puzzle, but we're now well into our journey of total fitness and there is so much to be optimistic about! Keep focused and your eyes on the prize. Now onto the next stage.

AGILITY - NOW THE FUN BEGINS!

AGILITY

It is the ability to move freely and easily.

Yet, its meaning goes beyond a dictionary definition. An agile person is fit, coordinated, supple, energetic, vibrant and athletic. It's the sort of person that most of us want to be but too few of us actually are.

The benefits of agility training for athletes are well established. It is the most effective way to enhance speed, alertness and coordination. In recent times, there has also been a growing realization of the huge benefits for non-athletes. To appreciate just how agility training can benefit you, let's take a closer look at how our muscles work.

Each of your muscles is made up of connective tissue, muscle tissue, nerves and blood vessels. All of these components coordinate to cause our limbs to move. Each muscle contains thousands of long, thin fibers. These fibers contain two opposing contractile proteins:

- Actin
- Myosin

These proteins repeatedly pull and release against each other. This causes muscular contraction which results in force. When we train the muscle, we enhance its ability to produce this force. This makes us stronger.

Speed, agility and quickness training is governed by what is called the stretch-shortening cycle. The cycle involves a combination of muscle lengthening (eccentric) and muscle shortening (concentric) actions. This acts just like a rubber band that is stretched out and then snaps back. When the eccentric action, such as dropping down into a squat position, comes before a concentric action, such as jumping onto a box, the force output of the concentric action is increased.

Agility training is built around increasing the ability of the stretch-shortening cycle. When you train the stretch-shortening cycle, you increase the connections between the muscles and the brain, allowing you to react faster and to exert more force. As a result, you are able to jump higher, change direction faster and react on the field more quickly.

AGILITY TRAINING BENEFITS

Weight Loss

Agility training is an excellent choice for weight loss. The nature of agility training makes it ideal to be performed in High Intensity Interval Training (HIIT) fashion. This is where you perform all-out effort on an exercise for a short period of time, followed by an even shorter active recovery exercise. You go back and forth between these moves for a set number of rounds.

Here's an example:

> *Stand in front of an agility ladder with a stopwatch in sight. As soon as the timer starts, jump both feet into the first rung of the ladder. Immediately jump them out to the sides of the ladder. Progress up and down the ladder in this manner, moving as fast as you possibly can. When 30 seconds is up, transition to a slow jog up and down the ladder for 10 seconds, before going back to the in-out jump movement for another 30 seconds. Continue until you have completed 8 rounds.*

This type of workout is extremely demanding. Though only taking a few minutes, it will burn a substantial number of calories while you are doing it. It will also bring on the enhanced post-exercise oxygen consumption (EPOC) effect. This will see you burning more calories while you are at rest for up to 38 hours after the workout.

Injury Prevention

Agility training is great for injury prevention. The enhanced balance, control and flexibility that is built as a result of agility training will massively improve your body's ability to maintain proper alignment and coordination when you walk, get up and maneuver your way around. If you stumble, you will be far more able to correct yourself before falling and hurting yourself. This type of training will also improve your posture and body placement, making you less likely to stumble in the first place.

Mind-Body Connection

Agility training, better than any other form of exercise, strengthens the connection between mind and body. As you consistently train yourself in agility movements, they will become second nature and you will develop the ability to move, coordinate, change position and weave without any conscious input.

Balance and Coordination

There is no better form of exercise to enhance your balance and coordination than agility training. By performing quick stop and start, and change of direction agility training exercises, you will be able to move with balanced coordination even when you are engaged in dynamic movement. As a result, your body will work together as a complete unit a lot better. You will also develop the eye-hand and foot coordination required for fast reflexes and reactions.

Better Recovery

Your ability to recover after intense exercise is a critical indicator of your fitness level. Agility training will allow you to build the heart and lung capacity to recover faster.

Faster Results

We've already mentioned how agility training, when done in HIIT fashion, can dramatically speed up your fat loss results. Agility training will actually get you fitter faster across the whole fitness spectrum. The non-linear movement involved with agility training brings into play many of the muscles that are not involved when you perform straight line training.

AGILITY TRAINING APPLIED: PLYOMETRICS

The most effective way to improve your agility is to do some form of plyometric training. Also known as ballistics or jump training, plyometrics involve explosive movement, jumping and quick lateral movement.

When it comes to people over the age of 40, the idea of jumping around may not sound very appealing. After all, their joints and bones are not as limber as they once were. That doesn't mean that they should avoid plyometrics, however. It simply means that you need to approach it smartly.

Smart plyometrics starts with an evaluation of whether you are ready for this form of exercise. A simple test is to take hold of a resistance band and stretch it overhead. From here squat down to full knee bend and then raise straight back up.

If you experience any movement limitation or discomfort while doing this move, you should continue to improve your mobility before you move into plyometric training.

You should also have a base level of strength through your glutes, hamstrings and lower back muscles before you begin plyometric training. You will strengthen these areas through your strength training. I suggest doing at least 12 weeks of strength training to build a foundation of strength in these areas before you introduce plyometrics into your routine.

When you decide that you are ready to incorporate plyometric training into your overall workout plan, I recommend adding them to your routine 1-2 times per week. Because plyometrics involves a lot of effort and requires a strong mind-muscle connection, I do not suggest doing them after your strength training sessions when you are already exhausted from your resistance workout. Performing plyometrics as a stand-alone workout will allow you to give the workout the justice it deserves.

Here is a Plyometric workout that will allow you to improve your agility safely while also increasing your explosive power.

Plyometrics Workout

- Skipping - 2 minutes
- Box Jumps - 60 seconds
- Broad Jumps - 30 seconds
- Skater Jumps - 30 seconds

Skipping

Don't worry if you can't skip - it is a learned practice. Just take it slow and try to build up the number of skips you can do without getting caught up in the rope. Start with skipping on both feet. You can also mimic the exercise without a rope at first to get your endurance up.

Box Jumps

Start with a very low box (less than 12 inches high). Begin with your feet shoulder width apart. Load your body by hinging at the hips, squatting down slightly and swinging your arms back. Now explode up onto the box jumping with both feet lifting at the same time. Land on both feet shoulder width apart into a slight squat and follow through with your arms. Step back down onto the floor and repeat.

Broad Jumps

Begin with your feet shoulder width apart. Load your body by hinging at the hips, squatting down slightly and swinging your arms back. Now jump forward explosively with both feet lifting at the same time. Land on both feet shoulder width apart into a slight squat.

Skater Jumps

Stand with your feet shoulder width apart. Now transfer your weight onto your right leg and lift your left foot off the floor and drop your hips slightly. Now jump to your left by pushing explosively off your right foot. Land on the left leg keeping your knee soft. As soon as you land, reverse the movement to jump back to the right. Try to spend as little time as possible in contact with the floor. Continue this back and forth movement until your time is up.

Agility Ladder Training

After 3 months of doing the above beginner's plyometric training program, you will be ready to add in agility ladder training.

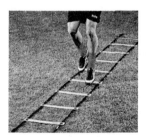

The Agility Ladder is an excellent investment to enhance your agility training. It consists of a rollable ladder made of plastic and canvas that is usually between 10 and 20 ladder rungs long.

Here is a 5 move agility ladder workout...

Agility Ladder Bunny Hops

With both feet together, bunny hop between each rung of your ladder, making light, quick touches in each square with the balls of your feet. When you reach the end rung, swing round and come back again. Imagine that the ground is hot, so that you make the quickest ground contact possible.

Single Leg Hops

Hop down the length of the ladder on one leg, then come back hopping on the other leg. Limit your ground contact to the balls of your feet, moving as quickly as possible. Your goal here is to maintain balance, not touching the rungs of the ladder.

Lateral Bunny Hop

Turn your body side on and bunny hop laterally (sideways) up and down your ladder. It is important to keep your upper body straight up and down on this one. If you lean to the side to build momentum, you will fall at the end.

Icky Shuffle

Start with one foot in the center of the first square and the other out to the side of the ladder. Now step the outside leg into the square, then the other leg out to the other side. Next, move the leg remaining in the rung up to the next square. The sequence is 'one-two-step-up'. Go as fast as you can, without touching your ladder.

Lateral Shuffle

Start with both feet outside the ladder. Step into the ladder with both feet and then out to the other side. As the last foot comes out of the ladder, tap it lightly on the ground and then straight into the next rung. Continue down your ladder. Your verbal cue for this move is 'one-two, one-two, tap and back'.

SUMMARY

Agility is your body's ability to move with grace, control and nimbleness. An agile person is able to adjust and recover, rather than fall and injure themselves. Working on improving your agility will allow you to move better; improve both your balance and recovery time and enhance your mind-body connection. It can also be a lot of fun! However, you need to make sure that your body is ready to take on the increased demands on the muscles and joints that come with agility training. Strength and mobility training will help you to increase your muscle and joint capability to meet these demands.

In the next chapter we will discover yet another foundation that is vital in our total fitness journey. This last physical foundation plays a huge role in every form of exercise we embark on…

8

ENDURANCE - DON'T STOP ME NOW!

NEVER GIVE UP!

It's a three word mantra that fathers pass on to their sons. We cling to it as quality of character, something to be esteemed and aspired to. It is exemplified in words like tenacity and perseverance.

But it all really comes down to endurance.

After all, when we run out of steam, our engine will stop - regardless of how much our mind wills it to keep going!

In this chapter, you are about to discover that the advancing years do not have to sap away at your endurance. In fact, I'm about to show you how you can enhance your get up and go, vitality and endurance every single day.

WHAT IS ENDURANCE?

Endurance is the ability to ward off fatigue for a long period of time. It is the product of a number of factors including:

- Aerobic Capacity
- VO_2 Max
- Lactate Threshold
- Muscle Strength
- Power
- Muscular Endurance

The main limiting factor for endurance is fatigue. Muscular endurance is also dependent on the ratio of fast and slow twitch muscle fibers that your muscles are composed of. Slow twitch muscle fibers have a higher endurance capacity than fast twitch fibers.

Endurance and stamina are often used interchangeably. The subtle difference between them is that endurance is all about the body's physical ability to go on. Stamina also includes mental fortitude.

There are two aspects to endurance:

- Cardiovascular
- Muscular

As we age, our endurance levels will naturally decline. From the age of 45 onwards, we will naturally lose an average of 5 percent of our endurance every decade. The reduction in size of the muscle fibers that occurs with aging results in lower levels of slow twitch muscle fibers. This will negatively impact muscular endurance. Natural loss of muscle function also negatively affects muscular endurance.

As we age, our bodies also become less efficient at using oxygen. Your cardiovascular endurance is dependent upon your body's ability to transport oxygen from the heart to the lungs and then onto the working muscles of the body.

The natural decline in maximal heart rate and VO_2 Max, and the maximum rate of oxygen that your body can use during exercise, also impact on endurance.

The reduced endurance that occurs as we age shows up with increased levels of fatigue. This is shown day to day by walking more slowly, running out of puff after checking the mailbox and having to sit down frequently to 'take a load off'.

Preserving endurance as we age is important for overall health and decreased risk of mortality. One study examined the association between the walking speed of a quarter mile distance and risk of mortality among 3,000 men and women between the ages of 70 and 79. Those with the slowest walking times (which was correlated to lower endurance levels) had the highest risk of death, cardiovascular disease and mobility limitation. 13 percent of the people were unable to complete the quarter mile distance as a result of fatigue.

REVERSING THE ENDURANCE TREND

The good news is that the natural age related endurance decline can be addressed, if not completely reversed. Training to improve your endurance requires that you improve both your cardiovascular and muscular endurance levels.

Improving Cardiovascular Endurance

Exercise to improve your cardiovascular endurance makes you breathe harder, working your heart and lungs and increasing the demand for oxygen. Examples are swimming, brisk walking, jogging, cycling and jumping rope (skipping). However, your cardio endurance program doesn't have to be confined to strict 'exercise' activities. Joining your local tennis/badminton club and playing a game of doubles twice a week or taking up dance lessons are also good options.

FITT-VP

The FITT-VP principle is a useful guideline to base endurance exercise upon. This acronym stands for:

- Frequency
- Intensity
- Time

- Type
- Volume
- Progression

Frequency

Frequency is about the length of each session and the frequency of the activity. If you are new to this type of exercise, start slowly with 10-15 minutes and then work progressively to meet the 150 minutes of cardiovascular exercise per week that is recommended by the American Heart Association. This total will include such other types of cardio exercise as the plyometrics you are doing to improve your agility but not your strength training.

Intensity

Training intensity is a measure of how hard your heart and lungs are working during your endurance workout. The higher the intensity, the greater the endurance-related benefits. Using a heart rate monitor is a good gauge of your aerobic intensity level. Calculate your maximum heart rate by subtracting your age from 220. The following table shows intensity levels as a percentage of maximum heart rate. To calculate your ideal heart rate at each level, multiply your maximum heart rate by the activity factor in the right hand box.

Intensity Level	% age of Max Heart Rate	Activity Factor
Very Light	55%	0.55
Light	60%	0.60
Moderate	70%	0.70
Vigorous	85%	0.85

Time

Time relates to the duration of the workout. Your training time should average about 30 minutes per day.

Type

Type should focus on exercises that involve large muscle groups. When it comes to training modes, cardio activities are grouped into the following four categories:

- Activities that can be done with minimal skill and fitness level (walking, cycling)
- Activities that are more vigorous but don't require a lot of skill (elliptical exercises, jogging)
- Activities that require a certain skill level (swimming, skating)
- Recreational sports (Basketball, tennis)

A well-rounded cardio program will select activities from each of these categories.

Volume

Volume is a measure of the total amount of exercise and is often expressed as total caloric output. Set an initial goal of burning 1,000 calories per week through cardio exercise.

Progression

Progression is the key to making continual improvement in your endurance level. By making your sessions slightly more intense you will be placing an adaptive stress on your cardio system that it will be forced to meet. Start to progress by increasing your training time. Then begin increasing your intensity level.

WARM UP

Spend 5 minutes before your endurance training session warming up. The following routine, which is a combination of dynamic stretching and aerobic warm up, is ideal if you are about to do an activity such as play a team game, ride a bike or go for a jog…

Start with a light jog for 1-2 minutes. If you are about to play a court game, cover the perimeter of the court. This will elevate your heart rate and get you breathing a little heavier.

Once you've got your heart and lungs moving a little, you're ready to lift the intensity slightly with a cardiovascular drill known as 'suicides.' This will lift your heart rate a little more while also stretching out your legs, back and arms. To do this drill, stand on the court sideline or facing a forward area of about 5 meters. Drop down into a sprint start position, with one leg back and the same hand touching the ground. Now jog forward to the centerline (about 2.5 meters), reaching down to touch it with your hand. Pivot and return to the sideline, and touch it with your hands. Now run the entire width of the court (around 5 meters) and touch the opposite sideline. Run back to the other side and again touch the baseline.

Do this forward suicide twice, moving at a jogging pace. Then, do it another two times but this time backpedal on the return each time.

Another great lateral agility warmup is called the Karaoke. This is a side to side shuffle with the added element that you cross one foot over the other with each step. Do this for two lengths of the court. The complexity of this action will engage your mind with your muscles, improving your proprioception and agility.

The aerobic warm up that we've just covered will get your heart rate up and increase your core body temperature in preparation for the game to come. Now you need to do some dynamic stretching in order to warm up your muscles.

Dynamic stretching involves moving your muscles through their full range of motion. Dynamic stretches often simulate the resistance moves that are part of the workout to come, such as doing bodyweight squats or lunges.

DYNAMIC STRETCHING ROUTINE

As well as the dynamic stretches we covered in the Mobility chapter, here is another 6 move dynamic stretching routine that will enhance your mobility ahead of your workout: Bear in mind, you can also mix and match ones from each chapter. It really comes down to how much time you have to warm up.

Hip Rotation x 5

Stand with your feet shoulder width apart. Now lift one leg into the air and rotate from the hip to perform a hip circle in a clockwise direction. After 5 rotations, reverse the motion to perform 5 anti-clockwise hip rotations. Now repeat on the other leg.

You may need to hold onto the tennis net or fence for balance while doing this dynamic stretch.

Knee Circles x 5

Stand with feet shoulder width apart and hands on hips. Now lift one foot slightly off the ground and begin to draw a circle in the air with your knee. The movement will be smaller than in the previous stretch. Perform 5 clockwise followed by 5 anti-clockwise circles. Now repeat on the other leg.

Ankle Circles x 5

Stand with feet shoulder width apart and hands on hips. Now lift one foot slightly off the ground and begin to draw circles with your ankles. This will be the smallest circle yet. Make sure to spread out your toes as you are performing your ankle circles. Again, perform 5 clockwise followed by 5 anti-clockwise circles. Now repeat on the other leg.

Shoulder Shrugs x 10

Stand with your arms extended out to your sides at shoulder level. Now shrug your shoulder blades up and down. This will warm up your shoulder joint and your trapezius muscles. Do this 10 times. Now, maintaining the same arms extended position, hold up your thumbs and then rotate at the wrist, supinate and pronate the hands up and down. Do not bend at the elbows as you do this. Do this 10 times.

SHOULDER CIRCLES

Stand in a neutral position with your arms level with your shoulders, extended away from your body. Keeping your shoulders relaxed, make small circles by rotating your arms backwards five times and then forwards 5 times.

Dynamic Swimmer Stretch x 10

Stand with your arms at your sides. Now bring them across your body to cross over and then extend them back to stretch out your pectoral muscles. In the extension, arch your back to feel the movement through your latissimus dorsi muscles. This action basically involves hugging yourself. Do this for 10 repetitions.

COOLDOWN

Cooling down after exercise or sport play is the most neglected part of being active. You've probably seen this yourself. How many people have you seen who take a few minutes to do some cool down stretches after the game? I'm betting that you could number them on one hand!

You need to be smarter than the majority of people when it comes to prioritizing the cooldown. Those few minutes can make a huge difference to how your body recovers and recuperates from your game or exercise session. A proper cooldown routine will help your muscles, tissues and joints to heal while also promoting enhanced blood flow to fast track nutrients and oxygen to your muscle cells. Once you have completed your main endurance session, you can simply walk for 2-3 minutes around the court, pitch or gym. This will bring your heart rate down gradually to your normal state. This will help to prevent issues like blood pooling, which we will cover later.

The rest of your cooldown will consist of static stretching.

Unlike some of the stretches in the Flexibility chapter that require lying on a mat, here is a sequence of 7 standing stretches that will take just a few minutes to complete…

Arm Stretch

Stand with your arms at your sides and your stomach pulled in, chest expanded and spine in a neutral position (not rounded). Clasp your hands behind your back and slowly lift your arms up, keeping your elbows straight. Hold for 15 - 20 seconds.

Triceps Stretch

Stand in a neutral position with your arms at your sides. Place your left hand behind your back so that your palm sits between your shoulder blades and your elbow points upward. Bring your right hand up behind your back and try to join hands. Hold for 15 - 20 seconds, then repeat with the other arm. You can use a towel to help you until you are able to join your hands.

Quad Stretch

Standing - Hold your foot at the lace part of your shoe (not your ankle), bring it behind your body and tuck your pelvis under so your tailbone is pointing at the wall in front of you (a posterior tilt). Try and get your heel to touch your bum without letting your knee swing out to the side. Hold for 15 - 20 seconds. Repeat with the other leg.

Neck Stretch

With your back straight and your chest lifted, clasp your hands loosely in front of you and relax your shoulders. Keeping your shoulders still, slowly lower your left ear towards your left shoulder. When you have tilted your head as far as is comfortable, hold the stretch. Repeat the stretch to the right.

Repeat this stretch 5 times each side.

Hamstring Stretch

Standing - With your feet hip width apart, place your right leg forward so your right heel is just in front of your left toe. Keeping your right leg straight, place your hands on your left knee and bend the knee. With a straight back, gently lean forward resting your weight on your bent leg. Hold for 15 - 20 seconds.

Overhead Stretch

Stand with your feet hip width apart, your back straight and your head in line with your spine. Lift your arms above your head as far as you can with your palms touching. Do not lean back and arch your lower back. Hold for 15 - 20 seconds. To extend this stretch further, ease your arms back slightly.

Standing Calf Stretch

Stand facing a wall and place your palms on it in line with your chest. Step your right leg back so that it is fully extended with your left knee slightly bent. Now lean forward to the wall, keeping your back foot completely on the floor. You should feel the stretch through your calf muscle. Hold the stretch for 15 - 20 seconds. Repeat on the other leg.

IMPROVING MUSCULAR ENDURANCE

Improving muscular endurance involves increasing the ability of your slow twitch muscle fibers to continue performing for an extended period of time. Very few activities work with your fast twitch or your slow twitch fibers exclusively but there are those which primarily work one of the two. Total fitness requires doing exercises that work both types of muscle fiber.

The following activities will primarily work your slow twitch muscle fibers...Steady state:

- Running
- Swimming
- Cycling
- Brisk Walking

Resistance training, such as the program that is detailed in Chapter 3 of this book, will work both your fast and slow twitch muscle fibers. Because our program includes both high and low rep ranges, you will activate primarily slow twitch fibers with reps higher than 15 and fast twitch fibers with reps below 15.

The current scientific thinking is that it is not possible to increase the number of either your fast or slow twitch muscle fibers. However, you can make them bigger and stronger with consistent training.

The workout protocols that we have already covered, including strength training and your cardiovascular endurance training will also cover your muscular endurance needs. As a result, you do not need to do any separate muscular endurance workouts.

SUMMARY

We have learned that both cardiovascular and muscular endurance are vital to your overall fitness. These types of training can be performed at the gym, at home, out in the park or at your local sports club. As with all exercise, the main ingredient is enjoyment. Take time to find what type of exercise you enjoy and are able to add into your lifestyle.

As we know, starting a new exercise program can be tough and seem daunting at the start, but having come this far in your fitness journey, you have discovered there are so many different components to keeping your body in great shape. Think of yourself like a chef, sprinkling these foundations into your weekly exercise routine. Remember you don't have to go all in right away - instead you should gradually build up all these 6 foundations week to week.

The 6 foundations we have covered so far are all based on physical activity but we still have one of the most important foundations left. This foundation is something that we deal with multiple times a day and can and will make all the difference to how you look and feel...

NUTRITION: YOU ARE WHAT YOU (CHOOSE) TO EAT

You are what you eat.

We've heard that statement so often that it has become cliché. But that by no means lessens its importance. You literally are what you eat. Your body is made from the following nutrients contained in food:

- Water
- Protein
- Carbohydrate
- Fat
- Vitamins
- Minerals

Nutrition is the science of how our bodies utilize that food. It boils down to two things:

1. Food's ability to produce energy to allow us to function.
2. The nutrients we need to build, maintain and repair the organs and systems in our bodies.

As a result, the food that we eat can have a transformative effect on our bodies. When you consistently eat 'unhealthy' foods (e.g. high fat, high salt, processed or sugary foods), your body will suffer. A lack of nutrients can, over time, cause your bones to become brittle, your gums to bleed, and your blood to carry insufficient oxygen to your cells. Too much of certain types of food, such as simple, high glycemic index carbohydrates, will pack unwanted body fat onto your frame. Being overweight or obese brings with it a whole host of related conditions, including cardiovascular disease, diabetes and osteoarthritis. On the other hand, eating foods such as vegetables, fruits, whole grains, beans, nuts and seeds, and lean protein have the benefit of providing the nutrients your body needs to function well without consuming too many calories. The simple fact is that not all foods are created equal. Later in this chapter, we will discuss these foods in more detail.

NUTRITION AND AGING

As we age, our nutritional needs change. Along with the changes such as muscle and bone density loss that we have already identified as affecting us as we grow older, our metabolism slows down and less stomach acid is produced.

Reduced metabolism means that we need to take in fewer calories, but a decrease in stomach acid means that we are less efficient at absorbing the nutrients in the foods we do eat. The micronutrients that have been identified as being difficult to absorb as we age are:

- Vitamin B12
- Calcium
- Iron
- Magnesium

This creates a Catch-22 like dilemma for people in their 40s and beyond; we need to take in *fewer calories* to get *more nutrients* into our bodies. This makes it essential that, if your goal is to achieve good health, body composition and fitness, you need to be more conscious of what you are putting into your mouth with every passing year.

Research has revealed another age related nutritional change - our ability to identify our body's signals for hunger and fullness are decreased. This leads to a decreased appetite as we age that can result in unhealthy weight loss and nutritional deficiencies. Our signals for thirst are also diminished as we age, which could lead to dehydration.

Coupled with the body's natural metabolic decline is the reduced level of activity that is normal with older people.

As a result, older people have a lessened need for calories to meet their energy needs. So, if you eat the same amounts of food that you did when you were younger, even if you were eating in a healthy manner, you are likely to pile on unwanted body fat. This extra weight will primarily deposit itself around your belly. This will be more pronounced among post-menopausal women as a result of reduced levels of estrogen.

MACRO & MICRONUTRIENTS

The nutrients in our foods are divided into two categories; Macro (large) and Micro (small). There are technically four macronutrients...

- Protein
- Carbohydrate
- Fat
- Alcohol

As alcohol is not essential for life, it is usually not mentioned with the other macros. It contains no minerals, fiber or vitamins, but does supply energy in the form of 7 calories per gram. These are what's known as 'Empty calories'

Micronutrients are the vitamins and minerals that are found in all foods, including herbs and spices. In fact, the micronutrient content of herbs and spices makes it a good idea to flavor your foods with them. This category also includes phytochemicals (found in plant-based foods) and zoochemicals (found in animal-based foods).

Micronutrients are essential to the body because they include the vitamins, minerals and chemical compounds that are vital to a healthy immune system and to the production of energy in the body. Minerals are also important for muscle growth and bone health. Eating a range of different foods will give you a full complement of micronutrients.

THE HEALTHY EATING PLATE

The question of how to get the right balance of macro and micronutrients for optimal health has been written about, debated and studied for decades. It can quickly become confusing for the average person who simply wants to know how they should be eating.

Governments around the world have been providing nutritional guidance to their citizens for decades. The USDA Food Pyramid is the most well-known set of food guidelines on the planet. The pyramid was designed in 1992, with its recommendations being eagerly adopted across the country. The Food Pyramid presented an illustrative representation of six food groups, with their position on a pyramid representing how frequently they should be consumed.

The only problem was that the advice it offered was dead wrong!

The food pyramid was based on the premise that all carbohydrates are good for our health. That is why carb-based foods such as breads and pastas formed the wide base of the pyramid. At the other end of the pyramid, representing its narrow tip, were fats, which were to be consumed sparingly.

As researchers identified the problems with the Food Pyramid, demands were made for an updated version. In 2011, the USDA Food Pyramid was replaced with a colorful plate shaped graphic known as MyPlate to represent the official US Dietary Guidelines. The plate, which is divided into segments to represent food groups, is easier to understand than the confusing food pyramid. MyPlate is divided into four sections:

- Fruits
- Vegetables
- Protein
- Grains

There is also a section, represented by a drinking glass, for water, dairy products and other drinks. Plus a small bottle which represents healthy oils.

Though it was a vast improvement on the Food Pyramid, MyPlate was by no means perfect. Harvard Health Publishing, a division of Harvard Medical School, responded to MyPlate by publishing its own Healthy Eating Plate. It offers more specific and more accurate recommendations for following a healthy diet than

MyPlate. In addition, the Healthy Eating Plate is based on the most up-to-date nutrition research, and it is not influenced by the food industry or agriculture policy.

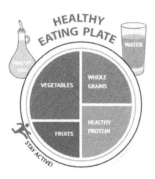

The Harvard Healthy Eating Plate recommends that your plate be made up of . . .

- Fruits and vegetables: ½ plate
- Whole grains: ¼ plate
- Protein: ¼ plate
- Healthy plant oils: in moderation

It also recommends that you drink water, coffee, or tea. You should skip sugary drinks, limit milk and dairy products to a maximum of two servings, and juice to just one small glass per day.

Finally, the figure running around the outside of the Healthy Eating plate is a reminder to stay active.

Let's break down these recommendations further.

VEGETABLES & FRUITS

Vegetables should form the basis of your diet. They are the most nutrient dense foods that exist, containing the vitamins, minerals and phytochemicals that your body needs to work at its best. Eating a variety of types and colors of vegetables and fruits provides your body with the mix of nutrients that it needs.

Here are some tips to help you increase your vegetable and fruit intake:

- Place fruit where you can see it - in a bowl on the kitchen counter or chopped up, fruit salad style in a bowl in the fridge.
- Go exploring down the produce aisle and regularly try new vegetables.
- Aim to get at least one serving each of the following daily; dark green leafy vegetables, red fruits & vegetables, legumes & peas, citrus fruits.

WHOLE GRAINS

Always choose whole grains over refined grains, which have been stripped of valuable nutrients during processing. There are three parts to the whole grain kernel:

- Bran
- Germ
- Endosperm

The bran is packed with fiber and contains the B-Vitamins, iron, copper, zinc, magnesium, antioxidants and phytochemicals. The germ is the core of the kernel and is a rich source of healthy fats, Vitamin E, B Vitamins, antioxidants and phytochemicals. The endosperm is the interior part of the kernel that contains the carbohydrate and protein.

Fiber is essential to healthy digestion and weight control. It slows down the breakdown of carbohydrates into glucose. This helps to balance out blood sugar levels and prevent sharp spikes in insulin release. Fiber also reduces unhealthy LDL cholesterol level and improves the movement of waste through the intestinal tract.

Emphasizing increased fiber intake over the age of 50 will help you to offset such issues as irregular bowel movements and digestive system upset. Having said this, it is important that your fiber intake is also high at a younger age. I myself have suffered from diverticulitis (an infection or inflammation of the intestines) in my early 30s. This was partly brought on by (amongst other factors) a fiber intake below the recommended levels.

You need to be careful when buying whole grains as some foods that are labeled as whole grain are not what they seem. The USDA provides the following 5 criteria for selecting healthy whole grains:

1. Whole grain' is the first ingredient on the ingredients list
2. Added sugars are not one of the first three ingredients
3. The word "whole" is included before any grain ingredient
4. A carbohydrate-to-fiber ratio of less than 10:1
5. The industry-sponsored Whole Grain Stamp

PROTEIN

Protein is the building material which the body uses to construct every part of you. There are more than 10,000 types of proteins in your body, and they are all made up of chains of amino acids. There are twenty amino acids, and nearly half of these (to be specific, nine) cannot be made by the body. These are called the essential amino acids and must be obtained from the foods we eat.

The UDS National Academy of Medicine recommends that adults consume a minimum of 0.8 grams of protein for every kilogram of body weight. However, for more active individuals this number needs to increase. The American college of sports medicine recommends a protein intake of 1.2 - 1.7 grams of protein per kilogram. In contrast, the International society of sports nutrition recommends 1.4 - 2 grams per kilogram. If we take both recommendations into account, we can come to a daily range of 1.2 -2 grams of protein for every kilogram of body weight.

This can understandably get confusing but it really comes down to what kind of exercise you're doing. Resistance based training - particularly activities like bodybuilding - will be at the higher end of 1.6 - 2 grams per Kilogram. On the other hand, more endurance -based exercises such as running or cycling would be at the lower end of 1.2-1.6 grams per Kilogram

The healthiest protein sources are fish, poultry, beans, nuts, red meat and cheese.

WATER

For millions of years, water was the only fluid that humans consumed. Our ancient ancestors only began drinking milk when animals were domesticated. Then followed the introduction of beer and wine. Today the amount of fluid choices is mind boggling, with the result that water, considered by many to be plain, tasteless and boring, is consumed far less frequently than it should be.

Your body thrives on water. In fact, every cell in your body soaks it up. 60% of your body weight is composed of water. To put that another way, if you're a 140-pound woman, 84 of those pounds are water!

The precise amount of water that you are carrying depends upon your body composition. Here's the water content of four major body constituents:

- Bone – 22%
- Fat Tissue – 25%
- Muscle – 75%
- Blood – 83%

We can divide the water in the body into two categories:

- Intracellular Fluid (ICF)
- Extracellular Fluid (ECF)

Around two thirds of the water in your body is intracellular, which means that it is contained within the cells. It contains a large amount of potassium and magnesium and a small amount of sodium and chloride. The rest of the water inside your body is found outside of the cell membranes. Of that amount, a quarter is contained within the vascular system, and makes up the plasma component of blood volume. The other three quarters is known as interstitial fluid, which is the fluid solution that surrounds your cells and connective tissue.

Without the right amount of water, your body will not function properly. Just take a look at what water does for you every second, without your realizing it:

- Regulates body temperature
- Lubricates joints
- Moistens tissues for mouth, eyes and nose
- Protects body organs and tissues
- Helps prevent constipation

- Helps dissolve minerals and other nutrients to make them accessible to the body
- Helps convert food to energy
- Carries nutrients and oxygen to the cells

Not only does it do all this, but the brain is composed of almost 75% water. Keeping the brain saturated prevents memory loss associated with aging. Drinking more water helps your kidneys and liver flush toxins out of your body. This will make your skin clearer and more radiant. Dehydration reduces the amount of blood in the body, forcing the heart to pump harder in order to deliver oxygen-bearing cells into our muscles.

Still not convinced how vital water is to your life? Then consider this:

You will still survive if you lose 50% of your body's glucose (energy), fat or protein.

You will die if you lose more than 20% of your body's water!

HOW MUCH WATER DO YOU NEED?

You may have heard the recommendation to drink 8 glasses of water each day. This is a good general guideline but may not be appropriate for everybody. The US National Academy of Medicine recommends a daily water intake of 13 cups for men and 9 cups for women. 1 cup is equivalent to 250 ml (9 oz).

Higher amounts will be needed by people who exercise or are involved in activities that cause them to sweat. The workout programs outlined in this book require that you increase your water intake. We recommend that you carry a water bottle with you throughout your workout and sip from it liberally.

You can determine whether your water intake is appropriate by looking at the color of your urine. Ideally, your urine should be straw colored, indicating that you are well hydrated. The darker your urine is, the less water you have in your body. So, if your urine is amber or honey colored, take this as a sign that you need to drink more water.

ELECTROLYTES

When we talk about electrolytes, we are referring to minerals that have the job of, among other things, facilitating the passage of fluids through cell membranes. Five key electrolytes are:

- Magnesium
- Sodium
- Potassium
- Chloride
- Calcium

Electrolytes also help to maintain a healthy pH level. This is a measure of how acidic or alkaline the body's solution is. When our electrolytes are out of balance, the body's fluids will tend to be overly acidic, which can cause a whole host of health problems.

It is vital to healthy body functioning that we have a proper balance of electrolytes. As with fluid intake, this balance depends upon the difference between electrolyte intake and electrolyte loss.

We lose electrolytes through urine and sweat. In order to replace them following intense exercise, researchers suggest taking a carbohydrate drink that is infused with electrolytes during and after the session.

You can help to maintain a healthy electrolyte balance by eating foods that are rich in electrolyte minerals. Here are five to get you started:

- Cheese (for sodium)
- Bananas (for potassium)
- Table salt (for chloride)
- Walnuts (for magnesium)
- Milk (for calcium)

CALORIC INTAKE

The fundamental reason that we eat is to supply the energy that our bodies need to function. If we don't supply enough of it through food, the body will draw upon its reserve energy source (stored body fat) to provide it. If we consume more than we need, the excess is stored on the body as reserve energy. Getting the right balance between energy intake and energy expenditure will largely determine whether we lose, gain, or maintain weight.

Energy from food is measured in calories. It is the amount of heat required to raise one liter of water one degree Celsius. When calories are consumed, they release heat, which is the energy that fuels us.

In the 19th century, a system was designed to affix a caloric amount to food. So, when we say that a food contains a certain number of calories, we have an indication of how much energy it will provide for the body. We are also able to determine the level of activity required to burn up calories. From this we can determine the caloric payoff for different types of exercise as well as the approximate number of calories the body requires each day to function.

A simplistic way to think about calories is in terms of a bank account. Your account is the store of calories in your body. Deposits are the calories you consume. Withdrawals are the calories you use up each day. If, at the end of the day, you have a surplus in your account, the number of stored calories will increase and you will gain weight. If you have a deficit, you will lose weight.

The reality is that it is more complicated than that. All calories are not created equal, the rate the body burns calories for energy is constantly changing, and the cascade of hormones throughout your body also play their part.

However, the law of energy balance gives us a good ballpark figure to how many calories we need to consume each day.

In order to work out your daily caloric requirement, you first need to know how many calories your body uses up each day.

Basal Metabolic Rate (BMR)

Your BMR is the number of calories that your body needs to sustain all of your body's functions while you are at rest. It accounts for 65 percent of your total caloric consumption. The other 35 percent comes from activity. About 80 percent of BMR is determined by lean body mass. The more muscle you have on your body, the higher your BMR will be. That is why one of the best things you can do to lose fat is to build muscle!

Working Out Your BMR

There are several ways to work out your BMR. One of the easiest and most reliable is what is known as the **Harris-Benedict Equation**. Although effective, this equation was updated in 1990 by Mifflin and St Jeor with around a 5% higher accuracy level. You could use either equation, but below I've used the more accurate **Mifflin and St Jeor** calculation.

An important fact to note before you begin is that this equation only works with metric units. If you know your weight in pounds and height in feet, you will need to convert these to kg and cm, respectively, before you begin.

Men:

BMR (kcal/day) = (10 x weight (kg)) + (6.25 x height (cm)) - (5 x age (years)) + 5

Women:

BMR (kcal/day) = (10 x weight (kg)) + (6.25 x height (cm)) - (5 x age (years)) - 161

Let's run through the equation with the example of a 70kg woman who is 60 years of age and 167 cm tall. Note, it's important to keep the brackets in, otherwise you will end up with a squiffy result!

BMR = (10 x 70) + (6.25 x 167) − (5 x 60) − 161
= **1283 calories per day**

This tells us that this woman needs to take in 1283 calories each day just to stay alive. But that doesn't account for any physical activity. To work out what out her caloric maintenance level is, we need to multiply the BMR by an activity factor as follows:

Exercise Level	Activity Factor
No Exercise	1.2
Exercise 1-3 times per week	1.375
Exercise 4-5 times per week	1.55
Exercise 6-7 times per week	1.725
Very labor-intensive job	1.9

Our 60-year-old woman exercises 1-3 times per week. So her activity factor is 1.375.

We need to multiply her BMR by that activity factor:

1283 x 1.375 = 1764 calories per day

Now is the time to do these calculations for yourself to know exactly how many calories need to be put into your body to maintain your current body weight. Once you know that number, then you will be able to adjust to burn body fat every single day.

Use the appropriate formula above to work out your BMR.

My BMR = _____ calories

Now multiply that figure by your selected Activity Factor to get your Caloric Maintenance Level.

My Caloric Maintenance Level = _____ calories

This is the number of calories you need to consume per day to maintain your weight. If you want to change your weight, there is one final step...

To lose body fat, subtract 500 calories per day.

To add lean muscle, add 500 calories per day.

Now we know about our ideal caloric intake and how to build a healthy and varied food plate, let's take a look at how you could apply this in your daily life.

SAMPLE DAILY MENU

Before Breakfast (½ liter water)

Breakfast

Cinnamon Apricot Breakfast Couscous

---

3 CUPS SKIM MILK, ONE 2-INCH CINNAMON STICK, 1 CUP DRY WHOLE-WHEAT COUSCOUS, ½ CUP DRIED APRICOTS, CHOPPED ¼ CUP RAISINS, 5 TEASPOONS BROWN SUGAR, PINCH OF SALT, 4 TEASPOONS CANOLA OIL

1. Pour the milk into a medium saucepan and drop in the cinnamon stick. Heat the milk over medium-high heat until small bubbles form around the edges. 2. Remove the saucepan from heat and stir in the remaining ingredients, reserving 1 teaspoon of brown sugar. 3. Cover and let the couscous stand for 10 to 15 minutes, or until the couscous absorbs the liquid. Remove and discard the cinnamon stick. 4. Sprinkle the remaining teaspoon of brown sugar on top to serve.

OR Poached Egg on Toast with Avocado Mash

2 MEDIUM POACHED EGGS, ½ AN AVOCADO MASH, 1 SLICE WHOLEMEAL TOAST, 5 CHERRY TOMATOES, HANDFUL OF SPINACH, WATERCRESS AND ARAGULA MIXED SALAD, TABLESPOON EXTRA VIRGIN OLIVE OIL, SQUEEZE OF LEMON JUICE

1. Boil the water with a squeeze of white wine vinegar for the eggs, mash the avocado into a bowl, cut the cherry tomatoes in half. 2. Put the toast on and poach the 2 eggs for 2- 2 ½ minutes on a medium heat. 3. When the toast is done, spread the avocado on the toast and place the tomatoes on top. 4. When the eggs are done place them on some kitchen towel to soak up the water. 5. Add the salad on the plate and drizzle with lemon and extra virgin olive oil, take the eggs off the towel and place on the plate, season with salt and pepper.

Snack

Apple + handful of walnuts or almonds

Lunch

Tuna salad with capers & olives

10–12 OUNCES CANNED TUNA (1–2 CANS) IN WATER, DRAINED ¼ CUP DICED CELERY, 3 TABLESPOONS FRESH LEMON JUICE, 2 TABLESPOONS CHOPPED ALMONDS, 2 TABLESPOONS RINSED AND CHOPPED CAPERS, 1 TABLESPOON EXTRA-VIRGIN OLIVE OIL, 1 TABLESPOON CHOPPED FRESH DILL SALT AND FRESHLY GROUND PEPPER

1. Flake the tuna with a fork into a mixing bowl. 2. Add the remaining ingredients except the salt and pepper, and stir until well combined. Season with salt and pepper. 3. Serve on wholemeal toast and/or a bed of greens.

Snack

2 tablespoons hummus with 8 baby carrots

Dinner

Italian Herbed Lamb Chops

> 2 TABLESPOONS EXTRA-VIRGIN OLIVE OIL, 1 TABLESPOON MINCED GARLIC, 6 BONE-IN LAMB CHOPS 1½ INCHES THICK, SALT AND FRESHLY GROUND PEPPER, 2 TABLESPOONS WHOLE-WHEAT FLOUR, 2 TABLESPOONS PLAIN BREAD CRUMBS, 1 TEASPOON DRIED OREGANO, ¼ TEASPOON DRIED THYME, ½ TEASPOON DRIED ROSEMARY
>
> 1. Heat the olive oil and garlic in a heavy skillet over medium-low heat. 2. Season the lamb chops with salt and pepper. 3. Combine the flour, bread crumbs, and herbs in a shallow dish and dredge the lamb chops to coat. 4. Arrange the chops in the skillet and cook for 5 to 7 minutes on each side, or until lightly browned, flipping every 3 minutes. 5. Let the chops rest in the skillet for 3 to 4 minutes before serving. Serve with your choice of green or red vegetables, legumes & peas, sweet potato mash.

Dessert

Simple Lemon Sorbet

> 1 CUP WATER, ¾ CUP SUGAR, ¾ CUP FRESH LEMON JUICE
>
> 1. Whisk together the water and sugar in a saucepan over medium heat. Stir until the sugar dissolves. Remove the sugar water from the heat and set aside. 2. Whisk in the lemon juice, then cover the mixture and chill it until cold. 3. Pour the mixture into a shallow pan and freeze it for 1 hour. Stir the mixture, then refreeze it until it is solid. 4. Just before serving, break the sorbet into pieces and blend it smooth in a food processor.

OR Easy Greek Yogurt

> 150g GREEK YOGURT, HANDFUL MIXED BERRIES, SPRINKLE OF MIXED SEEDS AND WALNUTS, DRIZZLE OF HONEY
>
> 1. Scoop the yogurt into the bowl. 2. Add the berries, walnuts and seeds on top. 3. Drizzle the honey...easy!

SUMMARY

As we have discovered in this chapter, nutrition is just as important - if not more so - than my other 6 foundations of total fitness. Consider that we eat 3-5 times a day, and there is temptation everywhere! Every few hours, we have to make decisions that can affect the way we look and feel. Luckily, we can use the simple Healthy Eating Plate to keep us on track. We now know about the key macro and micronutrients that are essential to keep us fit and healthy, and how we may need to adapt our nutrition to account for our changing metabolism as we grow older.

Digging deeper into nutrition requires another book in itself but when it all comes down to it, the vast majority of us do have the ability to change the way we eat for the better with willpower, controlled portions and a consistent routine. The good news is, life is all about balance so do enjoy treating yourself in moderation - and when you do, make sure you enjoy it!

We've been on a real journey together over the course of this book! We have now covered all 7 of my foundations of total fitness, and you should be feeling confident and motivated to get started with your new lifestyle. The best version of you is yet to come! Our final chapter will walk us through warming up and cooling down - vital for our preparation for, and recovery from, exercise.

10

WARM UP, COOLDOWN AND RECOVERY

WARMING UP & COOLING DOWN

Warming up and cooling down before and after an exercise session is something that we all know we should be doing. Yet, very few people give it the time and attention that it deserves. Many don't warm up at all, simply throwing themselves into the thick of their workout. You might be able to get away with that sort of recklessness in your teens or your 20s, but certainly not in your 40s or beyond.

Unless you ingrain the habit of gradually increasing your body's readiness for exercise you will suffer the consequences. Just think of what happens when you go to start your car on a cold, frosty morning. Don't you let it warm up for a minute or two before you take it out onto the highway? Doing so will allow its engine to run more efficiently. You, too, will operate more efficiently when you warm up before exercise.

When you are in a non-exercise state, around 20 percent of your body's total blood volume is contained in the muscles, with the balance being in our organs. When you warm up, you are able to transfer more blood from your organs to your muscles. That blood brings oxygen and nutrients into your working muscle cells. The blood then carries waste products out of the muscle cell.

The gradual increase of movement that occurs when you warm up also warms up your joints and lubricates them so they are primed for exercise movement.

Your warm up should feel quite easy. It is designed to get your body ready for the more intense work to follow. In a couple of chapters, we have already included specific warm up and cooldown routines that will gently prepare you for the workout and then return you to a state of inactivity.

It is important to also warm up thoroughly before you engage in any sport or active game activity. Whether you are playing pickleball or going for a jog through the park, it is vital that you ease your body into the activity. The one time that you skip your warmup because you're late or your team-mates are ready to get started is the one time that you will suffer an injury!

Cooling down is just as important. After intense resistance training or cardiovascular endurance like a long run or sprint session, your body is in a state of raised alert and it needs a small amount of time to gradually come back down to the safe zone. Think of it like driving a car at 70mph and all of a sudden slamming on the brakes! As you can imagine, this wouldn't be good for the car - or anything inside it.

When you are in a state of raised alert following exercise, your heart rate and breathing are both high as well as your blood pressure. A gradual return to your resting heart rate will help avoid dizziness or fainting. Feeling nauseous, dizzy or faint after exercise is usually caused by what is known as venous (blood) pooling. Blood is diverted to your muscles during exercise to ensure they have adequate oxygen to sustain the contractions required. This muscular contraction effectively squeezes your veins, which helps them to return your blood back to your heart against the pull of gravity. Venous pooling refers to the buildup of blood in your veins after the muscles in your limbs stop contracting following intense exercise, and normally occurs if you have not cooled down properly. Just a few minutes of rhythmic muscle contraction will be enough to help your blood return to your heart. Your blood pressure dropping will also assist the transition for blood from the lower extremities to return to resting flow patterns. This can all sound a bit scientific so here are a few easy things you can do to cool down:

1. Walk around the room or on a treadmill for 3-5 minutes.
2. Perform static stretches and if you have extra time, light foam rolling.
3. Focus on relaxing and breathing during the cool down. Remember you are winding down to go back to your day.

RECOVERY

Ensuring that you are fully recovered between exercise sessions is key to ensuring that you perform at your best and reduce your chance of injury. As they age, many people notice that their ability to recover is impaired significantly. In this section, we identify three things you can do to ensure that you maximize your recovery.

Sleep

Most people don't factor sleep into the recovery process. In fact, it is arguably the most important factor of them all. It is during this time that your muscles recover, repair and rebuild the muscle tissue that has been broken down during your workout. To achieve this, it needs around 8 hours of deep, restful slumber.

Obviously, when your body is resting through the night, it isn't being called upon to carry out all of the energy demanding requirements of the day. This allows it to concentrate on recovery and repair.

It is also during the hours that you are lying in your bed that a pair of extremely powerful hormones are released to do their work. These two hormones are...

- Human Growth Hormone
- Testosterone

As you probably already know, these two hormones are essential for muscle recovery, repair and growth.

Interrupted sleep is a key sign of overtraining, so it is important to monitor your sleep. If your sports watch or fitness tracker has a sleep monitoring function on it, be sure to make use of it. If you do create an overnight sleep debt prior to your workout, try to get a power nap after your training session. Even twenty minutes will be sufficient to make up the lost sleep.

For many active people it is a challenge to come to terms with sleep. They tend to view it as a sign of laziness. However, in order to optimize your training and recovery, you need to get out of that mindset and start to view sleep as an integral part of a smart training program.

Here are 7 hacks to ensure that your sleep is of the highest quality...

- Plan to get to bed at the same time every night and to wake up at the same time in the morning. I can't overstate the importance of routine!

- Maintain a dark, cool and quiet bedroom environment.
- Keep all forms of entertainment, including TVs, computers and tablets out of your bedroom.
- Avoid being active within 2-3 hours of bedtime. Spend that time winding down, both physically and mentally. An hour before retiring, turn off the TV, do your daily journaling and read a book.
- Don't consume caffeine after 2pm.
- Have a warm bath or shower about 90 minutes before bed. The hot water helps to lower your body temperature, which helps signal to the body that it's time for bed.
- Have a cup of herbal tea or hot milk an hour before going to bed.

Hydration

After reading Chapter Nine, you already know how important it is to drink water between workouts and while you are exercising. It's essential to replace lost body fluids and keep up your energy and strength levels.

But you shouldn't stop there. It is just as important to drink plenty of water AFTER your session has finished. After the workout your body is in a state of stress. Taking in a constant supply of water will lubricate it and help everything to work more efficiently. It will also allow the nutrients that your body needs straight after the workout (fast acting carbohydrates and protein) to get to the cells much faster.

Nutrition

In the previous chapter, we discussed the importance of a balanced diet for total fitness. I also outlined a suggested plan to hit your nutrition goals as outlined by the Healthy Eating Plate. However, if you are working out on a given day, you also need to consider the timing of your meals. About 90 minutes beforehand (120 minutes if you are swimming) you should have a whole food meal. This time window will give your body plenty of time for digestion before the added stress of your workout kicks into play. By the time you start your exercise, the nutrients will be coursing through your bloodstream in order to provide the fuel you need to move your muscles.

That pre-workout meal needs to contain a lean protein source and some slow release carbohydrates. Choose an easily digestible lean protein such as fish rather than red meat. The slow release carbs will give your muscles a constant energy supply over the next couple of hours. A great choice would be a large baked sweet potato, a palm sized chicken breast and broccoli.

Your workout will deplete the glycogen stores in your liver. Replace it by having a couple of bananas in the hour or so after your session.

CONCLUSION

In the introduction to this book, I made the rather bold claim that getting weaker, less conditioned and feebler as you age doesn't have to be your future lot in life. I told you that you don't have to conform to society's template of aging; that you could, in fact, become fitter, healthier and more agile with each passing year. In our journey from there to here, we have plotted our way through the roadmap to achieve those outcomes. This final chapter brings all of that information together to show you exactly how to implement it into your life.

So, let's recap and summarize our journey together. We began by taking an eyes wide open look at what happens to our bodies when we age. We discovered that our hearts become less efficient at pumping blood around our body, our bones become less dense, our muscles get smaller and weaker, our key hormones change in their output levels, our sleeping patterns change, our metabolism slows down, and we become fatter!

But…and this is the crucial point – we also learned that, though we may not be able to reverse all of the effects of aging, we can most definitely slow them down.

The key to thriving, rather than just surviving, as we age is summed up in the single word 'fitness'. We found out, however, that fitness is a far more holistic, encompassing concept than most people consider it to be. In fact, total fitness incorporates the following 7 foundations, that we can consider like the foundations of a building…

- Strength
- Flexibility
- Mobility
- Stability
- Agility
- Endurance
- Nutrition

We then began drilling down on each of those 7 foundations.

Strength training, we discovered, is a key to reversing the effects of aging. At that point, I made another bold statement (you may be starting to see a trend here). That statement bears repeating…

No matter your age or ability now, you NEED to take up

strength training and perform it consistently over the course of the rest of your life. It is never too late to start and, as soon as you do, your body and your mind will start to reap immediate benefits.

You were then provided with a basic sample strength training program that divided your body into two halves (upper and lower/core), so that you were working your upper body one day and your lower body and core the next.

We then introduced the aspect of mobility and provided you with a 3-part mobility drill to incorporate into your strength training warm-up. It comprised:

- Myofascial tissue massage to release and loosen muscles
- Dynamic stretching
- Mobility drills

Static stretching was brought in as a key component of your post-strength workout cooldown. This will, not only make you become more flexible, but will also help avoid injures and muscle soreness in the coming hours and days post workout.

We learned that stability exercises are a vital component in helping to prevent falls and avoid imbalances. We learned that the two aspects of stability that we need to train are active stability and passive stability, and looked at strategies to achieve these. We also looked at specific exercises to improve the stability of the core, lower limbs, lumbar spine, and shoulders.

When it comes to the next important fitness foundation - agility - we identified plyometric training as an ideal way to enhance that aspect of fitness. A four move plyometric workout was provided, with a more advanced agility ladder sequence as an agility training progression.

Endurance training, the sixth foundation of total fitness, involves two aspects: cardio and muscular endurance. Increasing your cardiovascular endurance can be achieved with swimming, brisk walking, jogging, cycling, and rope jumping. Playing active games you enjoy with your friends and family are also great ways to improve your cardio endurance. To enhance your muscular endurance, you should perform high repetitions on your strength workouts, in the 15 plus rep range. These have already been built into your strength training program.

The final foundation of total fitness that we discussed was nutrition. We identified the Harvard Healthy Eating Plate Model as a healthy, complete and balanced model to follow.

The Healthy Eating Plate promotes:

- A wide variety of vegetables and fruits
- A variety of whole grains
- Limited refined grains
- Healthy lean protein options like fish, poultry, beans and nuts

- Healthy oils, such as olive and canola oil for cooking, and on salads
- Plenty of water, supplemented by coffee and/ or a glass or two of milk daily

Let's now bring each of the 6 movement aspects of total fitness together into a weekly plan. Remember that your mobility drill and flexibility work bookend your strength training as the warm up and cooldown routines. You can however also add mobility drills into your main workout, as they can be done in between your resistance sets while you recover. It can get boring just waiting for the next set of weights and watching the clock tick, so doing a set of Cat Cows or Fire Hydrants in between your squats or bench press exercises can be very time efficient.

Below are two different example weekly routines that incorporate all 6 aspects in slightly different ways.

Weekly Total Fitness Plan 1

Mon	Tues	Wed	Thurs	Fri	Sat	Sun
Mobility Drills	*Mobility Drills*	Agility Training	*Mobility Drills*	*Mobility Drills*	Cardio Endurance	**Rest**
Strength Upper Body	**Strength Lower Body**	Stability Drills	**Strength Upper Body**	**Strength Lower Body**		
Plus: 5-10 mins Static Stretching	*Plus:* 5-10 mins Static Stretching	*Plus:* 5-10 mins Static Stretching	*Plus:* 5-10 mins Static Stretching	*Plus:* 5-10 mins Static Stretching	*Plus:* 5-10 mins Static Stretching	*Plus:* 5-10 mins Static Stretching

Weekly Total Fitness Plan 2

Mon	Tues	Wed	Thurs	Fri	Sat	Sun
Full Body Resistance Exercise & Mobility Drills	Stability Drills & Corrective Exercises	Full Body Resistance Exercise & Mobility Drills	Agility Drills & Corrective Exercises	Full Body Resistance Exercise & Mobility Drills	Cardio Endurance	Rest
Plus: 5-10 mins Static Stretching	*Plus:* 5-10 mins Static Stretching	*Plus:* 5-10 mins Static Stretching	*Plus:* 5-10 mins Static Stretching	*Plus:* 5-10 mins Static Stretching	*Plus:* 5-10 mins Static Stretching	
	Optional Cardio: Brisk Walk- 30 mins **or** Steady Jog- 20 mins		*Optional Cardio:* Brisk Walk- 30 mins **or** Steady Jog-20 mins			

We've now come to the end of the book, but this is just the beginning of your journey. All that remains now is to put what you have learned into practice. We all have different weekly routines and work schedules, so my advice is to incorporate these 7 foundations in a routine that you are able to be consistent with, alongside a healthy eating regime.

And that is perhaps the greatest challenge of them all.

You see, the majority of people who purchase fitness books get to this stage, end up with a head full of potentially life changing knowledge and then do…

…Nothing!

Procrastination and familiarity lead them back to their old way of doing things - you know, the very pattern of eating and non-activity that led them to buy the book in the first place.

So, the question before you now is this...

Are you going to revert back to the old, familiar, but body diminishing ways of old?

OR

Are you going to accept the challenges that have been presented before you, embrace the workout challenge and start thriving as the years advance, turning back the ravages of time and giving your body the respect it deserves?

...the choice is yours.

EXERCISE APPENDIX

Decline Dumbbell Press

Set an exercise bench to a 30 degree decline. Grab a pair of dumbbells and lie down on the bench. Extend your arms above you so that the dumbbells are over your lower chest. Slowly bring the dumbbells down to your torso. In the bottom position your elbows should form a 90 degree angle to your upper arms. Push back up to bring the dumbbells together in the top position.

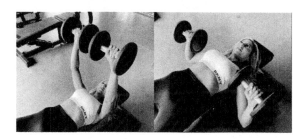

One Arm Lat Pull In

Place a seat in front of a cable pulley machine. Set the pulley on the highest setting and position the bench a few feet in front of the machine. Now sit side on to the machine and reach up to grab the cable with your closest arm. Adjust your position until your arm is at a 30 degree angle.

From this starting position, pull in and down until your elbow is down to hip height. Focus on fully contracting and extending your lats throughout the movement. See picture in chapter 3.

Shrugs

Hold a pair of dumbbells at arm's length with your palms facing into your thighs. Now, without bending the elbows, shrug your shoulders up and back in a circular motion.

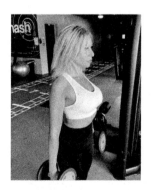

Cable Side Lateral Raises

Set the pulley on a cable pulley machine at hip height. Stand side on to the machine and grab the cable in your outside arm. With a straight arm bring the cable out and up to shoulder level. Slowly lower and return. See picture in chapter 3.

Cable Front Deltoid Press

Place a seat with a 90 degree upright a few feet in front on a double cable pulley machine, facing away from it. Set the pulley at hip height (when seated on the bench). Grab the handles and sit on the bench. Start with your hands by your sides with your elbows slightly behind your torso, palms up. Now push your arms forward and up to full extension in front of your body but do not lock your elbows. See picture in chapter 3.

Rear delt cable extension

Stand facing a cable pulley machine and about 3 feet away from it with the pulley set to eye height. Hold each handle but with the opposite hand so your arms cross over. Pull your arms out to the side then back behind your body squeezing your shoulder blades together. Slowly bring back to start position. See picture in chapter 3.

Cable Torso Rotation

Stand side on to a cable pulley machine and about three feet away from it with the pulley set at hip height. Grab the handle in both hands with arms extended in front of your body. Now rotate from the hips to twist away from the pulley machine. Return and repeat.

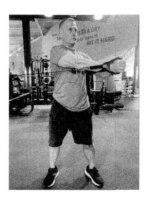

Cable Crunch

Place a seat with a back support about three feet in front of a cable pulley machine and facing away from it. Set the pulley to its highest setting. Place a rope handle on the cable. Now grab the handle with both hands and sit on the seat. The rope handles will now be at the side of your head. Crunch down to full contraction and then back to full extension.

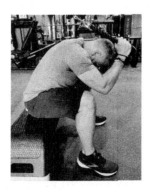

Seated Torso Extension

Sit on a seat with a light dumbbell held against your chest. Now round your spine forward to full contraction and then arch back to fully extend the lower back muscles. This is the same movement as the cable crunch but the resistance is operating in the other direction.

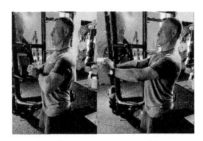

Cable Squat

Set the cables on a double pulley machine to the lowest setting. Face the machine and grab the handles stepping back a few steps. Try to stay upright as you squat down to a full squat. The weight should prevent you from falling back. Push through the heels to return to the start position. See picture in chapter 3.

Goblet Squat

If you are using a dumbbell, hold it vertically. Stand with feet shoulder width apart. Leading with your hips, lower your body into a squat keeping your feet flat on the ground. Keep your elbows inside your knees and go as low as you can maintaining a neutral spine (straight back and neck) Push through with your heels and stand tall without leaning back.

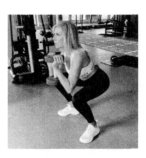

Glute kickback machine

Position your forearms on the machine pads and grip the handles. Maintain an engaged core and neutral spine. Place the arch of your foot onto the footpad and make sure your knee is in line with your hip. In a smooth motion, kick back to extend your hip and knee then squeeze your glute. Do not lock out your knee. Reverse the motion slowly with control.

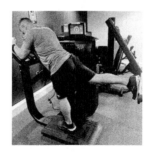

Seated Leg Curl

Position yourself on the seated leg curl machine at your local gym. Keep your hips, knees and toes in line. Pull down on the leg pads with your hamstrings to full contraction and then slowly release.

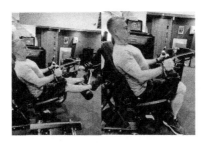

Seated or standing Calf Raise

Sit on a seated calf raise machine at your local gym. Position your feet on the footrest across the balls of your feet. Raise up on your toes to fully contract the calves. Now lower down below the level of the footrest to extend the calves completely. If you do not have a seated calf raise machine, you can do a standing calf raise using a kettlebell or dumbbell as seen here.

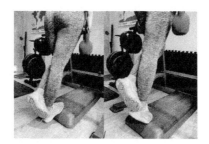

Alternative Dumbbell Reverse Lunges

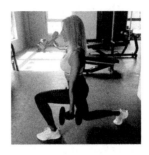

Using a mirror for this helps from a side view. Standing, take a large step backward with your right foot. Lower your hips so that your left thigh (front leg) becomes parallel to the floor so your left knee is directly above your ankle. Your right knee should be bent and in line with your torso pointing toward the floor with your heel lifted. Return to standing by pressing your left heel into the floor and bringing your right leg forward. Alternate legs.

Alternate Dumbbell Curl

Stand with a pair of dumbbells in your hands at your sides with palms facing your sides. Supinate your wrist as you curl the weight up to shoulder level. Be sure to keep your elbow in at your side and not to use momentum. Reverse the motion and repeat with the other arm.

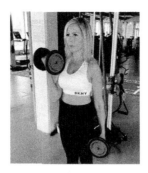

Decline Dumbbell Triceps Extension

Lie on a decline bench set to a 30 degree angle with a pair of dumbbells held above your head at full arm extension with your palms facing each other. Now bend at the elbows to bring the dumbbells down to the side of your head. Reverse the motion, being sure to keep your elbows in at your sides.

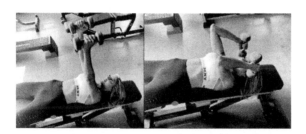

Barbell Wrist Curl

Sit on a bench with your knees together and a barbell in your hands. Place your forearms on your thighs so that your wrists and the weight are over your knees. Roll the barbell down your fingers to full extension and then curl the wrist up to full contraction. You can also do this with a dumbbell as seen below.

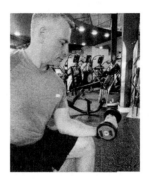

Barbell Hip Thrusts

Sit on the ground with a bench behind you. Keep your knees bent and hip width apart. Hold a barbell resting below your hips. Use a pad or towel for comfort. Lean back so your shoulder blades are on the bench and position the bar in the grove of your hips. Drive your hips up lifting the bar. At the top position your knees should be at 90°, with your body forming a straight line. Pause at the top of the lift and squeeze your glutes together, then lower your hips slowly. Start with no weight for higher reps.

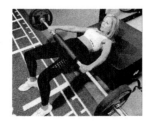

BREAKING BAD EATING HABITS

3 CRUCIAL STEPS TO HELP YOU STOP DIETING, INCREASE MINDFULNESS AND CHANGE YOUR LIFE - AT ANY AGE

INTRODUCTION

> "We cannot solve our problems with the same thinking we used when we created them"
>
> — ALBERT EINSTEIN

Here we go again.

You're about to get started on the diet that will finally propel you to your fat loss goals. At the same time, it will balance out your nutritional deficiencies, cure your gut problems and maximize your energy levels. You've been here before, of course – but this time, it's different. You're determined and failure is not an option! It will require a lot of pain, dedication and sacrifice, but you're up to the task – there will be no more cheating, quitting or excuses.

But you will fail.

Just like you have failed every other time, you've followed the traditional diet-based method to weight loss. The raw truth is that it doesn't matter how determined, dedicated or devoted you are if the foundation is flawed. And the foundation upon which the western world bases its weight control and healthy nutrition guidance is seriously flawed. That's why we are in the midst of an obesity epidemic that is threatening to drown us all in a sea of fat.

The way we eat is not dictated by science, logic or nutritional expert guidance. We may think it is but we're fooling ourselves. The real drivers of what we put into our mouths are deeply ingrained habits that begin to form during our first year of life. By the time we move out of our parent's house and set up on our own, our way of eating, the times, quantities, food selections, amounts, and speed of eating are cemented into our routine. Even if we come to the realization that some of those habits are not good for our health, our efforts to change them will be sabotaged. That's because those lifetime nutritional habits are not just part of our conscious being – they are also deeply ingrained into our subconscious.

Your subconscious mind is like the 90 percent of the iceberg that sits below the water. Even though you may not be consciously aware of it, the subconscious is the controller of everything you do. It will give a measure of freedom to the conscious mind, but as soon as you try to overturn deeply ingrained subconscious habits, it will pull you back into line, doing whatever it can to disrupt your new way of doing things.

When it comes to food habits, the subconscious has a powerful ally. Eating, as you probably know all too well, has never been about simply supplying the machine which is your body with fuel in the form of calories. It is an intensely emotional experience. We eat in response to how we are feeling. When we're upset, we rush to the pantry for sugar-loaded comfort food. Then, when we're happy we celebrate with party food. Emotional urges work in tandem with our ingrained subconscious habits to ensure that whatever we do to get on top of our eating ends up a miserable failure.

So, does that mean that we should all throw in the towel, give up on the insane idea of getting healthy and resign ourselves to a forever fat future?

Well, you could do that - but there is a better way.

And that better way is what this book is all about.

It's the reason I have decided to add yet another book on nutrition to a saturated market. As a personal trainer, I work at the coalface of the nutritional nightmare every day. Most of the people I coach are confused, mystified and frustrated at all of the conflicting and nonsensical information they receive in answer to the seemingly simple question, "What should I eat?"

Helping you achieve optimal health through sensible nutrition matters deeply to me because I, like you, have found achieving the right nutritional lifestyle challenging. It is a journey we all go through in life and the destination has taken time and effort to reach.

Over my years of working with hundreds of clients, I have discovered that there are 3 fundamental steps to achieving nutritional success. Whether your goal is to lose body fat, build lean muscle, get rid of gut problems, achieve optimal energy and health, or a combination of all of these. Here they are...

> Step 1 – Identifying habits throughout our lives and understanding why these have manifested.
>
> Step 2 – Change our mindset and learn how to break those habits through self-reflection, honesty and mindful eating techniques.
>
> Step 3 – Implement practical knowledge solutions to provide you with a detailed basic education in nutrition., along with practical tips and meal ideas.

The book you are about to read is set out in harmony with those 3 steps.

Chapters 1-4 explore the habits that have shaped the way we eat. We will come to understand how our upbringing and parental habits can shape not only our eating habits from a young age but also from pre-birth. Societal issues that help shape bad habits and that we use as excuses not to change will also be uncovered. We will also explore how aging and stress affect the way we eat. In this section, you will also discover why the diets that you may have been relying on in the past will never work - in fact, they will actually make you fatter!

Chapters 5 and 6 are where we begin to implement practical solutions so that you can break out of the eating habit trap. You will discover how to change your mindset, so you are able to create new rules that are guilt-free and easier to maintain a healthy lifestyle.

Our final section, Chapters 7-9, presents a treasure trove of practical solutions. You will learn of the importance of food as energy, as well as the role of hydration and recovery in combating issues like stress that can lead to bad habits. I will also present a no-nonsense, easy to understand grounding in nutrition, macro and micronutrients so you can feel confident going forward. We conclude with a bunch of ideas, tips and recipes to help you form better eating habits.

By the time you reach the end of this book, you will finally have the solution to the problem that has been sabotaging your efforts to get on top of nutrition. You will have gained the knowledge to overcome bad eating habits, ditched the dieting dilemma, optimized the way you eat with newer, better habits, and changed your life forever.

STEP ONE. IDENTIFYING HABITS

1

PRE-BIRTH NUTRITION, PARENTAL AND SOCIETAL INFLUENCE

"It isn't where you came from. It's where you're going that counts"

— ELLA FITZGERALD

NUTRITION DURING PREGNANCY

We have known for a long time that the foods we give our children and the messages we expose them to have an impact on their adult nutritional habits. Recent research, however, has revealed that parental influence on the way we eat goes back further than we ever expected. In fact, even before we take our first breath, the choices that our mother makes about what she puts in her mouth have an effect on us.

A 2008 study that was published in the journal *Science News* showed that poor nutritional choices made by pregnant women could put their baby at risk of developing long-term, irreversible health issues. These include obesity, increased HDL cholesterol concentrations and increased blood sugar levels. The study showed that the effects were more pronounced on females than on males.

Not only does the baby's experience in the womb affect its future health, but it is a determining factor in all areas of life, including future eating habits. A long-term research program known as the Developmental Origins of Health and Disease showed that the first 1,000 days of an individual's existence, counted from the moment of conception, were hugely impactful on the life of that child. Poor nutritional choices on the part of the mother can negatively impact the developing baby's development of organs and hormonal and metabolic responses.

The first month after conception is considered to be a crucial window during which it is most important that the mother eats a healthy, balanced diet. Of course, many women are not even aware that they're pregnant at this stage. This is one reason why prospective parents would do well to plan for pregnancy, with the female partner eating as if she were pregnant as a normal state of being. Their partner can also help by adopting these habits as support.

Each of the organs of the human body has a critical period of development. If there is a lack of nutrients due to poor food choices by the mother, the organ will be compromised. For example, if the fetus is poorly nourished when the kidneys develop, fewer nephrons will be produced. Their job is to filter blood. For the rest of that child's life, he or she will struggle to perform that vital function adequately.

Healthy eating during pregnancy includes eliminating processed foods and focusing on nutrient-dense foods. Here are nine nutrients to focus on during pregnancy:

- Folate
- Vitamin C
- Zinc
- Iron
- Fatty Acids
- Calcium
- Vitamin B12
- Vitamin D
- Choline

Prenatal nutrition even has an effect on our genetic makeup. Our basic genetic structure does not change, but environmental factors can make changes to the way our genes express themselves. An example of this was seen in the Netherlands during the Second World War, when famine led to a large number of malnourished pregnant women. This resulted in an adjustment in the epigenetic process known as DNA methylation in the offspring. These genetic expression adaptations predisposed the babies to later metabolic problems, elevated blood sugar levels, increased body mass index and higher LDL cholesterol levels.

In the last couple of decades, obstetricians have become increasingly alarmed at a new trend - obese babies. To have a baby come out of the womb weighing as much as 12 pounds is no longer a rarity. Hundreds of babies are born every year in the UK who are classified as being obese; that means that they weigh more than 9 lbs, 15 oz at birth.

As a result of the increasing fatness of babies, more and more women are being forced to have caesarean sections because the baby is too large to come out of the womb.

While it is true that some of these obese babies have piled on the pounds because their mothers suffer from a medical disorder, the vast majority are due to mothers eating too much. According to Tam Fry of the UK National Obesity Forum, "It is believed that 82 percent of children who are obese will continue to be overweight. As they had the same kind of nutrition as their parents, there is a continual spiral upwards."

CHILDHOOD INFLUENCES

Every baby starts out drinking mother's milk. But after that, it's all where you happen to have been born. If your first breath took place on the plains of Tanzania, post-milk nutritional experience would kick off with bone marrow from wild game. If you were born in the Far Eastern Republic of Laos, that first food would be gelatinous rice that has been pre-chewed by your mother and transferred from her mouth to yours. If you happen to be a western baby, your first bite of solid food is likely to be powdered cereal from a packet or puree from a jar. Those foods that are introduced early are the ones that will likely ingrain themselves as part of our eating habits.

None of us are born with an inbuilt knowledge of how and what to eat. These things have to be taught by our parents. From them, we learn what foods satisfy our hunger and provide us with the energy we need to function. We also learn when to stop eating. In former times, parents exposed their babies to a wide variety of food choices. However, over the past hundred years, those food choices have become far more homogenous.

During the first couple of years of life, our parents are the main determinants of our food choices. But from then onward, that decision making has increasingly been overtaken by food conglomerates. From as early as 2 years of age, children are continually exposed to food companies that are pushing foods that are high in sugar, saturated fats and salt. The youngster then puts pressure on their parents to feed them those foods. The addictive nature of high carb foods soon kicks in and the kid is soon unable to go through the day without their 'fix'.

Meanwhile, the food companies are coming up with ever more inventive ways to cash in children's longing for foods that nurture unhealthy eating habits.

The realization that our adult eating practices are shaped by the habits we learn as children should give us pause to rethink some of the things we have been doing with our kids. Think about eating vegetables. When we feel the need to hide carrots or brussels sprouts in other, more tempting foods, we are sending a strong message to our kids. We are telling them that vegetables are bad. Is that really what you want your kids to think? I don't think so.

Children are like sponges. They are always watching, analyzing and making conclusions. They do it about food perhaps more frequently than anything else. While a lot of what the child absorbs is conscious - like what to eat, when to eat it and when to stop - a surprising amount is subconscious. This includes the idea that, while vegetables are necessary, they are like an unpleasant medicine that has to be tolerated and that the good foods (in the sense of delighting the taste buds) are what we reward ourselves with when we want to celebrate and what we comfort ourselves with when we feel depressed.

Our basic food preferences, such as sweet or salty flavors are genetically predetermined. However, these genetic predispositions are modified by experience during childhood. The influence of parents in this process is huge. Research has shown that certain parental practices, such as exerting too much control over what and how much the child eats can contribute to the child being overweight. In their attempts to prevent children from having access to junk foods and pressuring them to eat healthy foods, many parents cause a negative rebellious reaction that sees the child eating more than other children of those 'forbidden fruit' foods as they develop a little more freedom in their pre-teens and teens. This often led to the child becoming overweight. Researchers conclude that it is much better to teach children by good parental example rather than imposing restrictions on them.

In the family environment, there is a wide interplay of factors that affect a child's perceptions around food. These include:

- The weight of the parents
- The parent's personal food choices
- Portion sizes
- Amount and types of food available at home
- Frequency of eating out
- Time of consumption
- Temperature and smell of foods
- Eating at the dinner table vs in front of the TV
- Physical activity
- The use of food as a reward
- The use of food as a comfort

Often, for the first year or two of a child's life, the parents are very mindful of what they feed their youngster. But then, as mum goes back to work, life gets busier and, often other kids come along, pre-child eating habits are reverted to. Setting a good example to the young one takes a back seat to the practicalities of life.

Here are 9 bad eating habits that kids pick up from their parents:

1. Salting food before tasting it - excessive salt consumption is a big problem, leading to high blood pressure and water retention.
2. Eating too fast - eating on the run is one of the root causes of overeating. That's because we don't give our body time to realize that it is full before the next mouthful enters the stomach. As a result, we are teaching our kids not to listen to their hunger cues! Eating on the run also denies the ability to savor and enjoy the abundant flavors in our foods, relegating eating to a purely mechanical process.
3. Skipping breakfast - mornings can get pretty hectic, making it difficult to find time to prepare breakfast. If we skip it, we are modeling that same behavior in our kids. Then, when they turn up at school without having topped up their fuel supply, they will lack focus in the classroom. By 11 am, they'll be desperate for sugary carbs, which they'll usually find at the school vending machine.
4. Overnight snacking - midnight snacking is a surefire route to fat gain. Don't model it, even if

you think the kids are sleeping. Instead, stop eating at least an hour before bedtime.
5. Avoiding vegetables - there's more to vegetables than mashed potatoes and a token bit of lettuce salad. If you tend to avoid vegetables, your kids will too. Parents who experiment with the wide variety of vegetables on offer are more likely to have kids who enjoy things like beets, butternut squash and zucchini.
6. Using food as a reward - having a sweet treat every now and then is fine, but when we reward ourselves, or our kids, with carb-loaded foods, we are sending them a powerful message; sugary foods are the jackpot! That message will very quickly become embedded into their subconscious.
7. Large portions - many kids who become overweight don't do so as a result of eating 'bad'; the problem is that they are eating too much food. The size of dinner plates has increased 30% since the 1950s. With most peoples' tendency being to fill the plate, it's hardly surprising that we are eating a whole lot more calories nowadays. So, rather than loading a large dinner plate and then telling your child that they have to eat everything that's on it, go out and buy a set of smaller plates and allow the child's natural hunger cues to dictate when they stop eating.
8. Not drinking enough water - if your child only sees you drinking coffee, soda, wine or beer, they

are not going to be very inclined to drink water, no matter how much you harp on about it. Modeling high water consumption is one of the best nutrition habits you can instill in your kids.
9. Fast food reliance - When life gets hectic, it's easy to forego the kitchen and either order KFC delivered or pack everyone in the car and head down to your local burger joint. But, think about what you are teaching your kids. Fast food is the 'go-to' solution whenever you get busy. Imagine how much better your child will be prepared for adult life if he saw you meal prepping fresh food rather than simply pulling out ready to go meals from the freezer.

MEDIA INFLUENCE

I don't have to tell you that the media pushes unhealthy food on kids - they've been doing it for more than fifty years. Of course, food companies have to get their message out there, but that doesn't account for the fact that 97% of all food advertising is for what nutritionists consider to be unhealthy food. Food companies spend more than $2 billion every year directly pushing their message to children. That is $1.94 billion being spent annually convincing your kids to put stuff into their bodies that is bad for them!

Governments around the world have been very slow to regulate the marketing of unhealthy food to children. In

2006, the UK government took the lead by imposing statutory restrictions preventing advertising for foods high in fats, sugars and salts around programs that were created for children under the age of 16. As a result of this measure, by 2009, according to a UK Department of Health report, the annual expenditure for child-themed food and drink products fell by 41%.

Measures like this are positive. The problem, however, is that fewer and fewer kids are watching TV. They are all online. And the food companies have complete free reign to push their high sugar, high fat and high sodium foods on social media platforms. As a result, we see more kids spending more hours sitting on their butts staring at a screen that is constantly enticing them with bad food. And then we wonder why we are in the midst of a childhood obesity epidemic!

How does all of this screen time exposure to food affect us? A study out of the University of Pittsburgh School of Medicine showed that study participants who spent the most time on social media were 2.6 times more likely to report problems with body image and eating than those who spent minimal time in front of the computer.

Another powerful influence on eating habits, especially as children enter their pre-teen years, is peer pressure. Research shows that more than three-quarters of pre-teens will make food choices when eating out that are in line with the preferences of their friends. Contrast this with the 40+ age group, in which just 2.7 percent of people will make fast food choices as a result of perceived peer pressure.

The food marketers take advantage of peer influence by constructing marketing campaigns to make kids feel they are missing out or that they're not part of the 'in' crowd if they don't buy their food product.

WHAT ABOUT EATING DISORDERS?

Eating disorders such as anorexia and bulimia nervosa are the result of complex and poorly understood causes. Sexual and mental abuse, parental conflict, pressure from sports coaches and the influence of society's ideals of body shape have all been implicated.

The eating disorder sufferer falls into a cycle of depression and low self-esteem, which they express through an obsession with their weight. Once they start to link body image and eating with mood and self-esteem, a cycle of extreme dieting and or/ bingeing and subsequent self-loathing can result.

They may see weight loss as the solution to their problems and feel that exerting strict control over their diet will help them control their emotional difficulties. All eating disorders are potentially dangerous. Sufferers are unlikely to help themselves and often deny having a problem. Most treatments emphasize both nutritional and psychological counseling.

SUMMARY

By the time we have moved out of our parent's home and are out on our own, we have all developed the habits that are going to drive our nutritional future. Those habits are an amalgam of all the things we have discussed in this chapter. For many of us, the combination of prenatal nutrition, cultural differences, food company advertising, parental example, social media influences, peer pressure, and societal pressures to look a certain way have resulted in bad nutritional habits that have put us in a place where we do not want to be.

In our next chapter, we explore the effect that poor nutritional choices have on the aging process. After revealing how bad food choices can speed up the aging process, we then drill down on the key anti-aging foods you need to focus on helping fight the effects of aging.

2

HOW BAD NUTRITION AFFECTS THE AGING PROCESS

"My belief is that it's a privilege to get older. Not everybody gets to be older"

— CAMERON DIAZ

Many people dread the aging process. After the age of 40, they view each coming birthday as one more marker that their body is declining, the vitality ebbing away and the march toward the grave quickening.

Then there are others who have a completely different view.

As they progress into their 40s, 50s and beyond, they view themselves as getting better, stronger and more energetic with each passing day. They accept, of course, that they are not immune to certain age-related physical changes, but they are not ruled by them. In fact, they accept them as a challenge and look for ways to minimize their effect so that they can retain their youthful vigor and enjoy life to the full.

Often the difference between the two comes down to nutrition.

In this chapter, we break down what happens to the body as we age and how our nutrition choices can either exacerbate or ameliorate that process.

HOW THE BODY CHANGES AS WE AGE

Fat Accumulation

The older you get, the harder it is to lose weight. From the age of 30, your metabolism steadily declines. That means that your body burns fewer calories. So, even if your activity level in your 40s is the same as it was in your 20s, you will still have a much harder time losing weight. That's one reason why it's so important to make smart food choices as we get older.

Allergies

As we age, we may find ourselves becoming allergic to things that did not affect us previously. Dairy is one of the most common allergies to emerge in later life. Many people in their 40s develop lactose intolerance. Your body creates lactase, an enzyme that digests lactose. But, as you age, your body produces less lactase, which makes it difficult to break down the lactose in dairy foods. This can result in bloating, headaches, diarrhea, gas and skin breakouts.

Plaque Build-Up

As we age, a build-up of cholesterol tends to line the arteries, making it increasingly difficult for blood to flow correctly. This could result in a blood clot or even a heart attack.

Reducing Perspiration

The older you get, the less you sweat. Women experience this more than men as a result of menopausal hormone changes. Sweat glands shrink and become less sensitive.

Reduced Muscle Mass

All people lose muscle mass as they get older. The muscles also lose their elasticity. Age-related muscle loss is called sarcopenia. From the age of 30 onward, men will lose between 3-5 percent of their muscle mass every decade. Reduced muscle mass makes a person weaker and reduces their functional mobility.

Brain Shrinkage

As we age, certain parts of the brain shrink. The most affected parts of the brain are those associated with learning and complex mental activities. Communication between neurons in parts of the brain is also negatively affected by aging. In addition, reduced neural blood flow and inflammation impair cognitive function.

As a result of age-related brain factors, older people may find it more challenging to recall names or other familiar information, having difficulty multitasking and a reduced attention span.

Reduced Tooth Sensitivity

As you age, the nerves in your teeth shrink. As a result, not only do your teeth become less sensitive, but you may be unaware if you have dental problems such as a cavity. That's why it's important to maintain a schedule of regular dental check-ups as you age.

Skin Changes

As you age, your skin becomes thinner, loses fat and produces more oil. This results in drier and less elastic skin. The number of nerve endings in the skin is also reduced, which results in reduced skin sensitivity. Older people also have fewer skin melanocytes, which makes them more susceptible to the effects of ultraviolet radiation.

Hair Quantity and Quality

As we age, we lose hair pigment cells, known as melanin. That's why our hair begins to turn grey. It also becomes thinner on the scalp, more frequently with men than women. As we age, our hair follicles produce thinner, smaller hairs. In time, they may produce none at all.

Loss of Height

We begin losing height in our 30s. Over the course of a lifetime, men can shrink about an inch, while women may lose double that. Height loss is the result of changes in bones, muscles and joints.

Urinary Function

The aging process is not kind to the bladder. It becomes weaker with the result that, as we age, we need to visit the bathroom more often. Uncontrollable bladder issues are also common as we age.

Facial Changes

In our 20s, our facial skin is rich in collagen and firm. From our 30s onward, the effects of sun exposure become evident. These include sunspots, wrinkles and dark patches on the forehead, cheeks and chin. In our 40's, facial skin is much drier, with prominent lines and wrinkles becoming etched in place. Subcutaneous facial skin reduces, often unevenly.

Heart Health

As we age, the heart begins to slow down in its activity. At the same time, arteries become stiffer. This combination of factors puts increasing pressure on the heart. This may cause the heart muscle to become enlarged. This is a contributing factor to heart disease.

Reduced Taste

By the age of 60, you will lose half of your taste buds. That's a big reason that older people seem to enjoy sweet treats more and tend to add a lot of salt to their food.

Hormonal Changes

Menopausal hormonal changes affect both men and women. This can make older people more susceptible to such conditions as diabetes, lupus and arthritis. Menopause in men is called andropause and is characterized by a drop in testosterone production.

Aching Bones

The older you get, the more likely you are to suffer from aching bones. This is the result of general wear and tear on the machine that is your body. Bone density decreases as we age. This makes bones more brittle, which can lead to bone fractures. Osteoarthritis is an age-related bone condition.

Digestive Disorder

Around 40 percent of seniors suffer from an age-related digestive disorder. One of the most common is constipation. This is characterized by painful or infrequent bowel movements and hard, dry stools. Also common are slower muscle contractions in the digestive system, which causes food to move more slowly through the colon.

Older adults often take medication, which may cause digestive issues. After the age of 50, there is also an increased risk of developing polyps, which are small growths in the colon. Polyps may become cancerous.

Research reveals that 20 percent of seniors have a condition known as atrophic gastritis, which results in low levels of stomach acid. This makes it more difficult to absorb nutrients, especially Vitamin B12 and the minerals iron, magnesium and calcium.

CHANGING NUTRITIONAL NEEDS

As we age, our nutrition requirements evolve. In order to offset many of the natural consequences of aging that we have just examined, it becomes increasingly important to eat a more healthy diet. Here is a summary of the significant aging changes specifically related to nutrition:

- Low stomach acid makes it much harder to absorb nutrients
- Slower metabolism results in a reduced caloric need
- Taste sensation is compromised
- There is a reduced sensitivity to our sensations of hunger and thirst
- Digestive system disorders including constipation, urinary problems and bloating

These changes present a sort of Catch 22 situation for older people; they need to take in **more** nutrients to offset reduced absorption while at the same time consuming **fewer** calories. In order to achieve these apparently contradictory ambitions, it is vital to focus on nutrient-dense foods.

Age-related metabolic rate decline is the result of a combination of factors. One of them is the gradual loss of muscle mass that takes place as we get older. Muscles are 5 times more dense than fat. As a result, it requires a lot more energy to sustain. As you lose muscle, your metabolism will be reduced. Reduced activity levels also result in a slower metabolism.

Even if a person in their 50s or 60s were to have the exact same level of activity and the same amount of muscle as a person in their 20s, they would still have a lower metabolism. This was shown in a 2001 study conducted by the University of Colorado. However, this change will not be nearly as significant as when the older person does little exercise and does not control their diet. In the study, the older men burned 71.8 calories per hour compared with 73.8 for the younger men.

What this shows is that the two key lifestyle factors of exercise and controlled nutrition are the most important controllers of metabolism as we age.

Reducing caloric intake is especially important in aging women. That's because the hormonal changes that occur during menopause lead to a decline in estrogen levels that can result in belly fat storage.

In order to meet their nutrient needs while eating fewer calories, older people should focus on eating the following whole foods:

- Vegetables
- Fruits
- Lean Meats
- Fish

The most important nutrients that are needed as we age are Vitamin B12, Vitamin D, Calcium and Protein.

Taking in more protein will help to offset the natural decline in muscle mass that occurs with aging. A 2008 study followed the dietary habits of more than 2000 older people over 3 years. It was found that those who ate the most protein experienced an average 40 percent lower rate of muscle decline than those who ate less protein. Those who combined increased protein intake with a regular program of resistance exercise experienced an even more significant reduction in natural muscle mass loss.

Constipation is a common problem amongst the elderly population. In people over the age of 65, it is three times more common in women than in men. One contributing factor is the medications that older people are taking that have constipation as one of their side effects. In order to help alleviate this problem, older people should concentrate on increasing their fiber consumption. Fiber is digested by the body, passing through and helping you pass softer and larger stools.

There are two types of fiber:

- Soluble
- Insoluble

Soluble fiber is found in such foods as nuts, seeds, beans, lentils and some fruits and vegetables. Insoluble fiber comes from whole grains, vegetables and wheat bran.

The majority of foods that are high in fiber contain a blend of soluble and insoluble fiber. Insoluble fiber will provide bulk to your stools. It also flushes the waste through the bowels to form them into stools. Soluble fiber absorbs water to create a gel-like substance. That becomes part of the stool. This will promote greater passage of the stool through the bowels.

As we age, our bones naturally become weaker and more brittle. Increasing our intake of Calcium and Vitamin D is the key to offsetting these changes. Calcium will help to increase the bone mass, while Vitamin D will increase the body's enhancement of Calcium. That's important because older people have a reduced ability to absorb Calcium. Researchers believe that this is due more to reduced Vitamin D intake than any natural decline. Also, as the body ages, it does not produce as much Vitamin D.

In order to get more Calcium and Vitamin D, older people should include a rich supply of the following in their diet:

- Dairy products
- Green leafy vegetables
- Salmon
- Herring

Older people also need more Vitamin B12, also known as cobalamin. B12 is required for the manufacture of red blood cells and for cognitive functioning. Studies have shown that between 10-30 percent of people over the age of 50 have a reduced ability to absorb Vitamin B12. This vitamin is attached to proteins in food. Before the body can use it, it must first be detached from its proteins. However, reduced levels of stomach acid make this a problem for older people. That is why taking a Vitamin B12 supplement is a good idea for seniors. Eating foods that have been fortified with B12 is also beneficial, as the B12 contained in them is not bound to protein.

Good sources of Vitamin B12 are eggs, fish, meat and dairy products.

As we age, our sensitivity to the thirst sensation is reduced. Couple this with the fact that kidney function can also be compromised with age, and it's no surprise that many older people do not drink enough water. This reduces cell fluid levels. A direct effect of this for older people is that it is much harder to absorb the active ingredients in medications.

Getting into the habit of drinking one or two glasses of water before eating a meal rather than relying on the thirst sensation will help older people stay well hydrated.

Older people often experience a reduced desire to eat. Age-related decreased appetite can result in nutrient deficiencies and exacerbated muscle tissue loss. Research shows that seniors have higher levels of leptin, the hunger-suppressing hormone and lower levels of ghrelin, the hunger initiating hormone.

The reasons for reduced appetite as we age may include less sensitivity of taste and smell, medications that decrease the appetite and the loss of teeth.

People who have difficulty eating large meals should eat several smaller meals spaced throughout the day. Eating nutrient-dense foods such as eggs, avocado, nuts and yogurt is also important.

9 FOODS THAT OLDER PEOPLE NEED TO REDUCE

As we age, it becomes even more important to avoid the foods we know we should steer clear of at any age. Here are the top 9 foods to cut back on.

Ice Cream, Candy & Cake

Sugar ages the body faster than any of the natural age declines we've discussed previously. Regularly eating it in the form of ice cream, candy and cake result in those sugars binding with protein. This has a negative impact on skin collagen, with the result that your skin loses its elasticity and youthfulness. Sugar also results in tooth discoloration and tooth decay.

Sugar, of course, is also the main culprit when it comes to unhealthy weight gain. Using natural sugar substitutes such as stevia and experimenting with natural fruit alternatives to sweet desserts will help you control your sweet urges.

Alcohol

Monitoring your alcohol intake is important at any age, but as we age, it becomes more critical. A healthy liver helps to eliminate toxins from the skin and other parts of the body. Excessive alcohol consumption, however, has a detrimental effect on the liver. Toxins that would otherwise be flushed from the body by the liver accumulate under the skin. This can lead to a prematurely aged look to the skin, swollen eyes, wrinkles and acne.

Alcohol also dehydrates the skin. This reduces the elasticity of the skin, as well as leading to patchiness, uneven pigmentation and dryness. It also destroys tooth enamel, which results in unattractive staining.

You don't have to become a teetotaler when you hit middle age, but you should cut down your intake. Moderation, as with most things, is the key to an enjoyable, healthy and long life.

Fried Foods & Sushi

Fried foods and sushi are very high in salt content, which causes water retention. This makes the skin appear puffy and bloated. Seniors should cut down on pre-cooked and preserved foods which are salt-heavy.

A diet that is high in salty foods increases the risk of high blood pressure and heart disease. It can also lead to excess Calcium in the urine, which increases the likelihood of developing kidney stones. Too much salt in the blood can also reduce blood flow to the heart and the brain. This increases the risk factor for heart attack and stroke. Researchers at the University of Maryland School of Medicine have estimated that a 50 percent reduction in salt content in restaurants and processed foods would save an estimated 150,000 lives per year.

Studies have also found that a diet rich in salty foods such as salty fish also increases the risk of gastric cancer.

Processed Meats

Processed meats such as sausages, corned beef, salami and ham contain lots of salts, preservatives and sulfites. These chemicals are known to trigger skin inflammation and accelerate the aging process. Processed meat is also one of the leading causes of heart disease, high blood pressure and respiratory complications.

The high amount of sodium in processed meats also contributes to puffiness and dehydration in the skin.

Char-Grilled Meats

Charred meat contains pro-inflammatory hydrocarbons, which cause damage to the collagen in the skin. That's why it is important to remove char from your grill after using the barbecue. When cooking meat, be careful not to over-grill it, as doing so could lead to the formation of skin-damaging free radicals.

You do not have to give up on red and white meats, as they provide an excellent source of protein. Just be sure to choose the leanest cuts possible and not overcook them. Pair them with green leafy vegetables that are rich in antioxidants.

Foods that Contain Trans Fats

Trans fats are a form of saturated fat. A trans fat is created when a vegetable oil undergoes the process of hydrogenation. This is done to extend the shelf life of the food by causing the food to harden at room temperature.

Commercially fried foods, cookies, crackers and margarines all contain trans fats. Trans fats can make even unsaturated fats act like saturated fats. You need to avoid them at all costs.

Trans fats do not fold upon themselves in the way that other fats do. Unfortunately, this leads to an increased risk of coronary heart disease, cancer and many other chronic conditions. What's more, trans fats increase bad LDL cholesterol levels and lower good HDL cholesterol levels.

A high intake of trans fats has also been linked to an increased risk of Alzheimer's disease, lymphoma, liver cholesterol synthesis, and suppressing the excretion of bile acids.

Here are five foods that are high in trans fatty acids:

- French fries
- Margarine
- Fried chicken
- Onion rings
- Donuts

Spicy Foods

Spices can cause havoc with your pH levels. The skin's pH levels are particularly sensitive to spices. This will cause skin irritation and may cause acne outbreaks. Spicy foods will intensify skin blotches. People with rashes will usually experience outbreaks after eating spicy food, especially during menopause. During this period, the blood vessels become more sensitive and reactive. This increases the likelihood of damage to the blood vessels when you eat spicy foods.

Caffeine

Caffeine is a diuretic that depletes the body of fluid and moisture. This can cause dehydration of the skin, making it look aged and dull. If you have developed a sizable coffee drinking habit over your lifetime, try to switch to decaffeinated versions. Another strategy to reduce your caffeine consumption is to set the target of matching every cup of coffee with a glass of water. This will have the dual purpose of keeping your body hydrated and filling you up on healthy liquids.

Canned Soup

Canned soup is high in sodium, preservatives and added artificial flavors. All of these are bad for your body. As we've already discovered, excess sodium will dehydrate your body and cause water retention. This will result in puffy skin and more visible fine lines.

So long as you avoid the ready-made, canned variety, soups can actually prove an excellent, nutrient dense meal for anyone and particularly seniors who struggle to eat solid foods. A blender or food sieve is all that you need to turn everyday ingredients into a filling, healthy dish. Homemade soups have a distinct advantage over canned versions as they allow you to control the levels of salt and sugar, and to preserve nutrients that are lost in processing. Try pumpkin soup made with pumpkin, onion, nutmeg, a stock cube and some water. You could also substitute vegetables such as broccoli and carrots for the pumpkin.

9 FOODS THAT OLDER PEOPLE NEED TO INCREASE

Water

Keeping ourselves well hydrated is important at any age, but especially so over the age of 40. Your body is around 60% water, with the blood containing 90%. You should aim to consume about 2 L of water every day. The challenge as we get older is that our sensation for thirst decreases. That makes it all the more important to consciously think about meeting your daily requirements. Keeping up your H2O intake will regulate your body temperature, help you think clearly, flush toxins from your body and help your muscles to contract strongly.

Broccoli

Broccoli is a super vegetable with both anti-inflammatory and anti-aging properties. As well as being packed with phytochemicals and high in protein, it is also full of antioxidants to combat free radical damage. In addition, broccoli is an excellent source of fiber. Maintaining a healthy fiber intake will not only keep you regular but help to control your appetite. Broccoli is a rich source of

Vitamin C. Among its other benefits, vitamin C promotes the production of collagen to keep the skin looking vibrant. Broccoli is even good for your brain as it contains folate, Calcium and lutein, which have been linked to enhanced memory.

For maximum benefit, eat your broccoli raw. If you prefer to eat it cooked, steaming will best preserve its nutrients.

Blueberries

Blueberries have the highest antioxidant counts of all fruits and vegetables. In fact, they contain a special type of antioxidant called anthocyanins. These are responsible for the blue color of this berry and contain powerful anti-aging properties. They are great for improving heart health, reducing cholesterol, fighting obesity, and slowing down age-related brain functioning degeneration. They even help to prevent colds and flu.

Nuts

Snacking on nuts and adding them to your salads, oatmeal and smoothies is a great way to increase your healthy nutrient intake. Two of the best sources are almonds and walnuts. Almonds provide an excellent source of vitamin E, which allows your body to repair damaged skin tissue, keeps your skin hydrated and protects it from sun damage. Be sure to eat almonds with their skins, as that is what contains the vast majority of the antioxidants in this nut. Almonds have also been shown to help to reduce cognitive decline in seniors.

Walnuts are a great source of Omega 3 fatty acids, which have a powerful anti-inflammatory effect. They have also been shown to help reduce the risk of heart disease.

Watercress

In addition to providing an excellent source of hydration, watercress is extremely nutrient-dense. It is especially high in vitamins A, C, K, B1 and B12. It's packed with antioxidants to fight off oxidative stress. In addition, watercress boosts immunity, improves digestion and supports thyroid function.

Bell Peppers

Red and orange bell peppers are especially high in antioxidants. Red bell peppers have the highest vitamin C content, which helps to build collagen to keep your skin looking healthy. The bright colors of bell peppers are due to what are known as carotenoids. These contain powerful anti-inflammatory properties.

Bell peppers make a satisfying snack on their own, especially if dipped in hummus.

Spinach

Spinach is another vegetable that will improve your hydration while delivering a powerful antioxidant boost to your body. Just like red bell peppers, spinach is high in vitamin C. It's also an excellent source of vitamin A, which is great for hair health, and vitamin K, which helps fight off inflammation.

Avocado

Avocados are a genuine superfood. They contain healthy fatty acids that ward off inflammation in the body and promote healthy skin. They are also rich in carotenoids and vitamins A and E. These two vitamins will help to keep the skin looking youthful and nourished. The high levels of antioxidants and avocados make them among the best foods you can eat to counter the oxidative stress caused by free radicals.

Chickpeas

Chickpeas are an excellent source of protein. As we've discovered already, as we age, we need fewer calories but just as much, if not more, protein. Getting it through sources such as chickpeas is a smart way to go. They are very nutrient-dense and contain a high protein count for their calorie cost. As well as being a very good source of protein, chickpeas are also high in fiber, iron and copper.

Cutting back on red meat as your go to source for protein and increasing your intake of plant-based sources such as chickpeas, beans and legumes is a smart move for seniors.

AVOIDING WEIGHT GAIN AS YOU AGE

Many people gain weight as they age. However, research makes it clear that age-related weight gain is by no means inevitable. While the body's metabolic rate does slow down after the mid to late 30s, the main reason why people gain weight seems to be because they are not physically active and are eating too much food, regardless of how healthy that food happens to be.

For women, menopause also leads to changes in fat distribution. This is due to a drop in estrogen levels. At this time of life, fat begins to collect around the waist and on the stomach. By understanding that the body now needs fewer calories, you can make changes at the crucial time and prevent, or at least reduce, weight gain. Preventing weight gain will involve far less effort than trying to lose weight later on.

Try to stay as active as possible as you get older - exercise is still a major factor in a healthy life, helping to alleviate the symptoms of arthritis and increased joint mobility. In fact, you should be more active during middle age to burn off the extra calories that your slower metabolism is not using.

Identifying your specific nutritional needs and adapting your food intake accordingly is a lifelong commitment. If, for example, you become ill and are bedridden, the nutritional value of your food needs to be high, but your calorie intake requirements will be reduced as you are completely inactive. If you are short of time and find it difficult to include exercise or activity in your day, a similar adjustment should be made. Conversely, it is important to maintain a healthy weight and not let your weight fall too low as you age - evidence suggests that fractures associated with osteoporosis are more likely among thinner people.

SUMMARY

There is no denying that the body undergoes natural changes as we age, and not for the better. Here's a summary:

- We get fatter
- Allergies become more of an issue
- Plaque builds up on our arteries
- We sweat less
- We reduce muscle mass
- The brain shrinks
- Our teeth become less sensitive
- Our skin becomes thinner, less elastic and drier
- Our hair becomes less vibrant
- We get shorter
- The bladder becomes weaker
- Our heart activity slows down
- Our taste sensation is reduced
- Our hormonal activity changes
- Our bone density decreases
- We experience digestive system disorders

As we age, we need to adjust our nutritional habits in order to offset these changes. The essence of those changes is that we need to eat fewer calories but receive higher nutrient density.

In order to meet their nutrient needs while eating fewer calories, older people should focus on eating the following whole foods:

- Vegetables
- Fruits
- Lean Meats
- Fish

The most important nutrients that are needed as we age are Vitamin B12, Vitamin D, Calcium and Protein.

3

STRESS AND OUR GUTS

"Breath is the power behind all things. I breathe in and know that good things will happen"

— TAO PORCHON-LYNCH

Stress is something that we all live with. The change and uncertainty that we are faced with on a daily basis present us with unique physiological, psychological and physical challenges. Our body's response to those challenges is what we call stress. Its physical manifestations are increased heart rate, muscle tension, elevated blood pressure and either expansion or constriction of our lung capacity. These changes prepare us for what is called the 'fight or flight syndrome,' in which the body is on 'high alert' to respond to the crisis.

Not all stress is bad. A controlled level of stress primes us to perform at our best. It allows us to react quickly to danger or to give extra effort to a challenging situation, such as going into a job interview. However, ongoing stress can be detrimental to our health, our thinking ability and our ability to perform and recover from exercise.

Stress affects every part of the body. Adrenaline and cortisol are released by the nervous system, which causes increased levels of blood pressure, heart rate and glucose. Too many of these hormones flowing through our system can result in headaches, irritability and insomnia.

Stress causes the muscles of our body to become tense. This is a protective mechanism to stave off injury. However, muscle tension can result in aches and pains, tension headaches and muscular spasms. Our rate of breathing increases as we work to bring in more oxygen. This can cause shortness of breath and hyperventilation. Stress will also cause the heart to beat faster in order to transport oxygen and nutrients to the muscles and organs of the body.

Stress also affects the way that we digest food. As a result, an inordinate amount of stress can lead to both diarrhea and constipation. Cloudy thinking, mental confusion and rash decision-making may also result from too much stress. It can cause us to act in ways that are out of character with our normal behavior. We may become sharp with others, make cutting remarks or fail to follow through on our responsibilities.

Stress can also lead to weight gain. Researchers have identified cortisol as the primary culprit in stress-related weight gain. They have also found that weight gain from cortisol primarily accumulates around the waistline!

STRESS AND AGING

Recent research indicates that the most stressful years in our lives are between the ages of 40 and 54. One study revealed that meeting financial obligations was a greater concern for people in this age group than at any other stage of life. A quarter of people over the age of 40 were also going through the stress of a relationship break up. Other major stressors for people in the 40-54 age group were the financial pressures of raising children and putting them through tertiary education, along with trying to prepare a nest egg for retirement. Health problems related to aging were also found to be contributors to stress in this age group.

THE EFFECT OF STRESS ON YOUR GUT

Your body is home to around a hundred trillion microorganisms, each of which plays a vital role in the way your body looks and feels. Within your stomach lies an intricate complex of viruses, bacteria and fungi that are collectively referred to as your gut microbiome. It's also known as the Garden of Life. Just like any garden, your gut microbiome prospers when you look after it and deteriorates when you neglect it.

Since 2007, the Human Microbiome Project, a US National Institute of Health (NIH) research initiative, has examined the gut microbiome. In the process, more than a thousand species of microbes have been identified. The researchers have also identified the key jobs of your gut bacteria:

- It breaks down complex carbs
- It produces compounds such as vitamins B12, K, B3 and B6
- It produces short-chain fatty acids
- It strengthens the immune system
- It helps to detoxify the body
- It helps to protect the body from pathogens
- It modulates the nervous system

This is not an exhaustive list, but it is enough to give us an idea of the vital role the gut microbiome plays in orchestrating overall wellness. If you allow it to get out of sync, you will gain weight, opening yourself up to such complications as irritable bowel syndrome, heart disease and inflammatory bowel disease (IBD).

Recent research has shown your gut flora plays an essential role in weight control. It has been revealed that your gut microbes send fullness signals to your brain to tell it when to stop eating. In addition, the gut microbiome influences the vital balance between blood glucose and insulin levels. Your gut flora also controls your rate of metabolism.

All three of these factors – appetite control, blood glucose and insulin regulation and metabolism rate – are vital to weight control.

A large body of research makes it clear that stress has a major impact on gut health. The following gut issues have been directly linked to stress . . .

Inflammatory Bowel Disease (IBD)

A 2005 study that was published in *Gut* magazine concluded that chronic stress could increase the risk of relapse for people who suffered from IBDs such as Crohn's Disease and ulcerative colitis. The researchers identified a number of mechanisms by which stress impacts both systemic and gastrointestinal immune and inflammatory responses.

Irritable Bowel Syndrome (IBS)

A study that involved more than 600 people found that the ability to handle stress was a key indicator as to whether patients whose gastroenteritis caused campylobacter went on to develop IBS.

Gastroesophageal Reflux Disease

One study found that, even though there was no indication that increased stress increases the frequency of acid reflux, stress does lead to an increased perception of acid reflux severity.

Peptic Ulcer Disease

While researchers no longer believe that Helicobacter Pylori (H. pylori) is directly caused by chronic stress, there is evidence that stress leads to mucosal lining inflammation, which allows gastric juices to irritate the lining of the stomach.

HOW STRESS AFFECTS THE DIGESTIVE SYSTEM

If you've ever had to give a speech, you probably already know that stress affects your stomach. What we commonly refer to as butterflies in the stomach is a physical manifestation of this phenomenon. It occurs because the brain and the gut are in constant communication. Your gut contains around 500 billion neurons which are collectively known as the enteric nervous system. These are partly controlled by the central nervous system in the brain.

The enteric nervous system is located in the gastrointestinal lining that runs from the esophagus to the rectum. It regulates the following processes:

- Swallowing
- Releasing enzymes that break down food
- Categorizing ingested nutrients as either food or waste products

When we are under stress, each of these processes is negatively impacted. Specifically, stress may cause the esophagus to spasm, increase acid build-up in the stomach, cause a nauseous feeling and lead to diarrhea or constipation.

HOW YOUR GUT BACTERIA GET OUT OF BALANCE

Let's start by considering where gut bacteria come from.

When you were in your mother's womb, you had a sterile environment within your intestines. The microbiome that you begin life with is inherited from her. It is transferred during the time you pass through the birth canal, as well as when you are breastfed.

Apart from the gut, the female vagina is home to a large population of gut flora. Some of this vaginal fluid is swallowed by the emerging baby. These are the first of the trillions of gut flora that colonize your intestines.

Breast milk contains bifidobacteria, which is an important probiotic. It also boosts the development of biofilms that line the gastrointestinal tract.

Some fascinating research has highlighted just how critical this formative gut flora is to lifelong weight control. A 2013 study by Azad et al showed that children who were born by C-section have much lower levels of healthy bacteria in their gut. This makes them more susceptible to serious illnesses, including allergies, asthma, inflammatory bowel syndrome, celiac disease and Type 1 Diabetes. They also found that babies who were born by C-section are at a higher risk for developing obesity.

A really interesting extra fact to come out of this study (and others like it) is that the microbial imbalances that begin at birth can last for up to 7 years.

Obviously, you had no control over what happened back then. But there are a number of other factors that contribute to the state of your gut's bacteria. The most influential one is nutrition.

Everything we eat is digested and metabolized by the flora in our gut. It is obvious, then, that your gut flora is operating optimally. That means that it has to be fed the right way.

So, what happens to your gut microbiome when you consume the typical American diet?

Foods that are high in processed carbohydrates, sugar, trans fats and artificial additives are, not surprisingly, bad news for your gut. The end result is that they will reduce the overall biodiversity of your gut flora. As reported in the journal *Future Microbiology,* an adjustment in the biodiversity of your gut microbiome leads to fat gain.

There are other factors that influence the state of health of your gut flora. Antibiotics are major bad news for your intestines. And yet, we have become a nation of prescription drug addicts. And we've turned our children into antibiotic dependents as well.

Mirroring the alarming increase in childhood drug dependency has been a considerable increase in the rate of childhood obesity. The connection is plain to see. In fact, a study by Bailey, LC, et al., which was published in the journal *JAMA Pediatrics* in 2014, revealed that youngsters who were given a broad spectrum of antibiotics prior to the age of two were far more likely to become obese during childhood.

Our environment is another big influencer on our gut bacteria. Species of flora come into the body when we're rolling around in the playground, kissing the dog, or even swallowing dirt.

As you are no doubt well aware, the mollycoddling nature of modern society has transformed the environmental influencers on our children. They don't play in the dirt anymore. We've become so bacteria phobic that our children are not being exposed to the natural influencers that can help to shape healthy gut bacteria.

Studies have shown children who are brought up on farms, where they are interacting with farm animals and getting back to nature, have a healthier balance of gut flora. As a result, they get sick less often and are less prone to obesity.

So, the over-sterilized, cotton wool environment that has been thrust upon us – and that we have, in turn, thrust upon our children – has not made a healthier society at all. It has, in fact, done the opposite . . .

It has set the stage for an epidemic of ill health and obesity.

THE MOOD / FOOD CONNECTION

Your food and your mood are directly related to one another. Yet, the vast majority of people are oblivious to this vital connection. They become obsessed with treating the symptoms of negative moods and miss out on the underlying causes. Often that cause is tied up with what you are putting down your throat.

The degradation of soil over the last fifty years has dramatically impacted the nutrient content of foods. In fact, it would take six apples for you to get the same nutritional value of just one apple from fifty years ago. On the African continent, the soil is nowhere as depleted as America. As a result, their fruits and vegetables are far more nutrient-dense. The result is that people who live over there generally have better teeth and bone structure.

One of the most important minerals for the body is potassium. It acts as a physiological tranquilizer, in effect calming the nervous system down. Bananas are well known for containing potassium. A single banana will provide 400 milligrams of potassium. However, we need 4700 milligrams of potassium per day just to meet our minimum daily requirement. That equates to 7-10 servings of vegetables per day.

You need potassium for two key reasons:

- To calm down your heart rate
- To maintain stable blood sugar levels

The B Vitamins are also very important for mood regulation. When you are feeling stressed, you quickly use up the B vitamins. This causes you to become more anxious and nervous. The most important B vitamin, and the one that gets exhausted first when you are stressed, is Vitamin B1. The best source of Vitamin B replacement is nutritional yeast. This can be picked up from your local health food store. Add a teaspoon to your yogurt or protein shake every day. It will help to calm you down as well as assisting you to get a good night's sleep.

Calcium is another key mineral for mood regulation. It helps to calm down and relax when you are in a stressed state. Stress causes calcium to pass right through the body without getting adequately absorbed. If you decide to supplement with a calcium product, do not use one that is derived from calcium carbonate. Instead, go for a supplement that is derived from calcium citrate, cheese or plain yogurt.

Omega-3 fatty acids are vital for proper brain functioning. You should supplement with high-quality fish oil, taking in 1000 mg per day.

Iodine is one more important mineral for mood elevation. Iodine supports the thyroid, which assists with the cognitive functioning of the brain. The best source of iodine is from sea kelp.

Regulating Blood Sugar

The amount of sugar in your blood has a direct effect on your mood. If your blood sugar level is too high, you are going to experience brain fog, typified by memory loss and impaired cognition. When the level is too low, you will become moody and irritable.

The biggest influencer on blood sugar levels is your consumption of simple carbohydrates. By switching around some of your basic eating habits, you can make considerable improvements in your blood sugar stability and, as a result, your mood.

Most people have been eating a carb-based breakfast their whole lives. It is either built around cereal or toast. This surges sugar into your body first thing in the morning, causing your blood sugar level to go up and resulting in a less than optimal cognitive functioning. The body's response to this high level of blood sugar is to release more insulin from the pancreas in order to clear the blood out. This leads to overcompensation and suddenly, you do not have enough sugar in the blood. Now you become moody and, around mid-morning hungry for more carbs to get your blood sugar levels back up. When you do, the whole vicious cycle repeats itself.

Simply by switching from a carb-based to a protein-based breakfast, you avoid all of these problems. Make eggs a staple of your breakfast menu and you'll be taking in close to 20 grams of high-grade protein to support lean muscle growth throughout the day (an average egg contains about

6 grams of protein. And you needn't worry about the cholesterol in the yolks. Scientists have recently shown that there are no issues with up to eating 2-3 eggs per day.

You should also consider having a whey-based protein shake as a breakfast alternative. Look for a low-carb protein mix that contains whey isolate protein, as it will digest faster than other forms. A protein-based breakfast will help to stabilize your blood sugar levels right throughout the remainder of the day. Avoiding sugar is the most important thing you can do to improve your mood.

Hormones and Your Mood

Hormones have a huge influence on your brain, and therefore your mood. Serotonin is a pleasure hormone that makes you feel good. It acts as a neurotransmitter that sends messages to your brain. You can thus build up your serotonin levels through your diet. To do so, you can increase your consumption of foods that contain tryptophan, the amino acid which is the building block of serotonin.

The following ten foods are all high in tryptophan:

- Free-range turkey
- Flaxseed
- Buckwheat
- Wild fish
- Whey protein
- Bananas

- Eggs
- Sour cherries
- Free-range beef
- Dark chocolate

Cortisol is the stress hormone. It leads to anxiety and constant worry, where your mind is going at a hundred miles an hour thinking about negative things. Exercising and maintaining a clean diet that is free of junk food and simple carbs are two of the best strategies for keeping your cortisol levels down.

The following foods will help you to control your cortisol levels:

- Coldwater fish
- Walnuts
- Swiss Chard
- Eggs
- Dark chocolate
- Greek Yogurt
- Citrus Fruit
- Pumpkin seeds
- Spinach

Food and beverages to avoid to control cortisol . . .

- Alcohol
- Caffeine
- Low fiber carbohydrates

- Flavored yogurt
- Fruit juice
- Trans fats

STRESS & WEIGHT GAIN

Stress not only makes us cranky, irritable and frazzled; it also makes us fatter. Recent research has shown that stress-induced cortisol release leads to fat gain. Specifically, cortisol fat gain tends to collect around the middle of the body. A 2011 study found that women with greater abdominal fat had more negative moods and higher levels of life stress. The lead researcher, Elissa S. Epel, Ph.D., concluded that 'greater exposure to life stress or psychological vulnerability to stress may explain their enhanced cortisol reactivity. In turn, their cortisol exposure may have led them to accumulate greater abdominal fat.'

Conversely, when cortisol levels are lowered, abdominal fat levels come down. In another study, researchers from the University of California at San Francisco randomly assigned chronically stressed overweight and obese women to nine weekly sessions (lasting two and a half hours each) of mindfulness training and practice, where they learned stress reduction and awareness techniques. Additionally, the women in the mindfulness group were asked to meditate for thirty minutes a day. The control group received no mindfulness training. Although no diets were prescribed, both groups did attend one session about the basics of healthy eating and exercise.

Then, the researchers measured the participants' psychological stress, fat, deep abdominal fat, weight, and cortisol levels before and after the four-month study. The link they found was clear: when women's cortisol levels went down, so did their abdominal fat levels. Further, those with the most significant reductions in cortisol had the greatest reductions in abdominal fat.

The link between stress-induced cortisol levels and abdominal fat gain couldn't be clearer. Incorporating the mindful breathing technique can help you control stress and bring down your cortisol level.

STRESS & THINKING ABILITY

One of the most immediate effects of stress is to impact our ability to think clearly. Cortisol, the same hormone that causes abdominal weight gain, will alter the structure and function of the brain. Excess levels of cortisol cause overproduction of a neurotransmitter called glutamate. Too much glutamate is not good; in fact, it becomes a neurotoxin which causes free radical activity that can actually kill brain cells.

One of the most immediate stress-related cognitive effects is forgetfulness. Stress causes electrical signals in the brain, which weaken the memory. At the same time, the parts of the brain associated with emotion are enhanced. That makes us more likely to make rash decisions based upon emotion and less likely to follow through on our healthy lifestyle choices. In other words, when you're stressed, you are more likely to make the decision to ditch your workout and reach for a cookie instead!

STRESS' IMPACT ON METABOLISM

Have you ever noticed that your body doesn't seem to digest food very well when you're overly stressed? It's no coincidence. Stress and the stomach are unavoidably linked. That's because the portion of the brain that activates stress deactivates digestion. A part of the central nervous system called the autonomic nervous system (ANS) turns on the gastric processes in the stomach that allow us to digest food. The ANS also tells the stomach when to switch off. When our body switches into fight or flight mode, it switches off digestion. As a result, we experience gastric problems.

Cortisol is one of the key drivers that puts us into fight or flight mode. This hormone speeds up the breakdown of glucose and fat to provide the body with the energy required to respond to the emergency situation that it perceives when we are under stress. This results in an increased metabolism.

TOP 10 WAYS TO DEAL WITH STRESS

We can't avoid stress. It is the body's inbuilt device to help us to cope with what life throws at us. From the moment we crawl out of bed until the time we return to the covers, it is a constant that we have to contend with. So, removing stress from our lives is an unrealistic goal.

What we can do is to learn to better manage the stress that we encounter. For most people, stress is brought about when the events in their life are uncontrollable or unpredictable. Many people, in fact, define stress as being the time when they feel as if they have no control over their lives. Research has shown that when people learn to relinquish control over every aspect of their life, they feel less stressed.

Here are ten scientifically proven ways to more meaningfully manage your stress.

Stress Buster #1: Learn to Breathe

Learning to breathe correctly is the most fundamental thing you can do to reduce your stress levels and improve your overall wellbeing. Your basic life processes, such as your heartbeat and respiration, are controlled by your autonomic nervous system. For a long time, it was believed that we had no conscious control over its operation.

We now know that many aspects of the autonomic nervous system can be controlled by the individual. The way we control them is by breathing from the belly. The simplest and most direct form of stress management is to move from a shallow, stressed state of breathing into deep, belly breathing.

In learning to breathe again, you will be consciously thinking about your breathing - perhaps for the first time in your life. After a while, though, you'll no longer have to think about it. Deep breathing will become habitual. Until then, however, you will need to consciously make an effort to breathe correctly. You won't be breathing properly with every breath straight away and you shouldn't expect to.

Start by taking in deep breaths for 20 seconds every hour. Slowly increase until you are doing it for a minute at a time. After a week, you'll be up to 5 or 6 minutes every hour. At the end of 3 months, the old ineffective way of getting oxygen into your system will be a thing of the past. Your body will no longer be sputtering down the road on half a cylinder - you'll be cruising along on all 4 cylinders, with the hood down and the wind blowing through your hair!

How to Do It

Stand or sit comfortably. Now, take in a long, deep breath through your nose until the lungs are completely full and your chest is inflated. Hold this breath for 5 full seconds. Now, allow the breath to slowly leave your body. Be thinking about expanding and compressing the diaphragm as if it were an accordion on every inward and outward breath.

The Power of Nasal Breathing

Learning to breathe through your nose will make you a far more effective in-taker of oxygen. When you inhale through the nose, you will be taking the air more deeply into your diaphragm. Try it right now and you will be able to feel your diaphragm expanding. This expansion puts downward pressure on your abdomen. This has the flow-on effect of pushing air into the lungs and enhancing the circulation of blood and nutrients. This form of breathing is also more relaxing than mouth breathing.

Test Yourself: Breathe 100

Take in 100 nasal breaths in a row. Exhale through your mouth each time. Next, focus on breathing in with just your right nostril—breathe out through your left. After 100 breaths, swap sides. As a final nasal challenge, breathe in 100 times, holding for 10 seconds after each breath.

Sub-10: Your Breathing Goal

When you are breathing optimally, you will be taking in no more than 10 breaths a minute, ideally just seven or eight. Your goal is to achieve as many sub-10 breath minutes as possible in your day.

Breathing Exercise

The breathing method just outlined will allow you to dramatically improve the amount of oxygen that comes into your body. That's great moving forward. However, you still have to contend with a whole lifetime of ineffective breathing. The following breathing exercise will allow you to strengthen and maintain power in your lungs.

Do this first thing in the morning upon waking and again in the mid-afternoon (it will provide a caffeine-free way of overcoming the 3 o'clock slump!).

> Step One: Get comfortable, either standing or sitting.
> Step Two: Breathe in through the nose for 5 seconds. Feel your stomach pushing out as the energy-giving oxygen fills your lungs.
> Step Three: Hold for 20 seconds. Feel the oxygen circulating around your body as it gives life to your trillions of cells.
> Step Four: Repeat this process four more times.

When performing lung exercises, it is important to focus on inflating the lungs upward and outward rather than downward. Imagine that the intake of oxygen is about to lift you up and carry you skyward.

The Pay Off

Learning to breathe correctly will be frustrating and annoying to start with. But remember back to when you began to learn to ride a bike? That was frustrating. It was annoying. And it was probably painful. But you persevered. If you had given up, you probably wouldn't be whizzing around in a car today. Same thing with learning to breathe. In fact, there are at least 14 direct benefits that come with deep breathing:

- Enhanced toxin release

- Enhanced tension release
- Better clarity and relaxation
- Relieves emotional pressure
- Eases physical pain
- Increases muscle mass
- Strengthens immune system
- Enhances digestion of food
- Enhances nervous system functioning
- Strengthens the lungs
- Helps burn fat
- Boosts energy levels
- Enhances cellular regeneration
- Makes you happier

Stress Buster #2: Learn to Appreciate

Too often, we take life for granted. Yet, learning to appreciate what we have by seeing the good and the value in what we have right now is a key stress reducer.

It is very easy to fix our attention on all the things that are going wrong in our lives. It takes real effort for us to see the good, even though it's right in front of our faces. In fact, the very process of slowing down in order to 'smell the roses' is difficult for most people. The ironic thing is that it is this inability to slow down and appreciate the everyday little things that is a key stress contributor.

When you train your mind to think about the good things that you have, despite the negative curveballs that come your way, you can actually reverse the stress response.

Here is how you can purposefully implement the appreciation strategy:

> When you wake up in the morning, mentally review the things you need to do in the day and include on that list two things that you are grateful for.

> When you feel stress coming on, take two deep belly breaths. When you inhale for the third breath, let your mind focus on someone you love, a place you enjoy being at, or an act of kindness someone has done for you.

> Throughout your day, regularly focus on someone you love, a place you enjoy being at, or an act of kindness someone has done for you for up to 30 seconds at a time.

Stress Buster #3: Slow Down

Life is hectic. Everybody is in such a hurry to get from Point A to Point B and to move from one thing to the next. We have appallingly short attention spans and we have lost the ability to be patient and wait. All of those things are bound to bring on stress.

The simple act of slowing down is a fundamental skill that will make your life more relaxed. It is only when we learn to slow down that we truly get to appreciate the beauty of the lives that we live. Slowing down is not difficult, but making it a practice in your life can be. To succeed you need to work at it.

Start by taking notice of what you eat. Take the time to taste and savor your food. This eating with attentive care will help you to make smarter food choices and avoid weight gain.

You don't have to slow down all day long, but you should have an OFF switch that allows you to slow down when you want to. Slowing down will put less strain on your body and give you more energy as you go about your daily activities.

To instigate the slowing down process, simply tell yourself that you have all the time in the world. As you slow down, become totally absorbed in and focused on what you are doing. Doing so will not only reduce stress – it will make you a much better person to be around!

Stress Buster #4: Relax Your Muscles

When we get stressed, our muscles become tense. In fact, our bodies can become so used to this bunched-up feeling of tension that we are no longer able to relax, even when we aren't stressed. It is possible, however, to train the body to react in a relaxed manner to a stressful situation.

Stress brings about a natural tightness of muscle and restricted flow of blood to the hands and the feet. Tense muscles feel heavy, whereas relaxed muscles feel light. The interesting thing is that our muscles are the most relaxed immediately after they have been tensed.

Consciously tensing and relaxing is a skill that you can develop in order to alleviate stress. You can even do this while driving the car. Grip the steering wheel tightly and then relax your grip. You'll immediately feel how relaxed the muscles in your arms feel.

Here's how to apply this life skill . . .

> Before you go to bed, exercise, sitting at your desk or are stuck in traffic, take two slow, deep belly breaths. On the third inhalation, tighten your right arm from the shoulder to the hand.
> How this position for three seconds.
> As you exhale, relax the arm entirely and let it drop.
> Repeat with the other arm.

Stress Buster #5: Visualize Success

Visualizing success involves removing from your mind the negative images of failure that you have and replacing them with positive images of success. When you visualize success, your body will immediately relax and the body calms itself. In contrast, the practice that most people have of constantly feeding themselves negativity leads to stress.

To make success visualization work for you, think about an area of your life in which you are not successful. Now take three slow, deep belly breaths. Now build up an image of yourself succeeding at that activity. Next, describe to yourself what the image showed you about how to be successful at the activity. Ask yourself how success was different from the things you usually do. Now plan ways to implement that knowledge into your future performance.

Practice this process at least three times for every area of your life that you want to find more success in.

Stress Buster #6: Appreciate Yourself

The majority of people out there see a glass as being half empty, especially when that glass is themselves. They fixate on their failings without giving any credit to themselves for their good points. Learning to appreciate yourself will lead to an immediate reduction in stress along with greater self-contentment.

Learning to appreciate yourself essentially comes back to self-talk. The vast majority of our self-talk is negative. We tell ourselves that we are a failure, that we are not as good, not as attractive or not as smart. Life coaching guru Zig Ziglar referred to this as 'stinkin' thinkin'.

It is your job to banish 'stinkin' thinkin' from your life. When a negative thought enters your mind, quash it and replace it with a positive one. Every day, think of at least one thing that you did that was helpful or something that you were good at.

Be confident in the person that you are. Know your identity and values and be proud of them. If they are out of step with the mainstream, don't feel the need to apologize for them. Appreciate yourself, be proud and confident, and you will project an aura of confidence that will be attractive to others.

Stress Buster #7: Change Behaviors

You've probably heard of the quote which is most often attributed to Albert Einstein that says that 'the definition of insanity is doing the same thing over and over and expecting a different result.' Often the behaviors that cause stress are things that we repeat over and over again. Changing those behaviors is a key to stress relief.

To make this stress buster a success, you need to identify the things that aren't working in your life and stop doing them. Then, implement a new strategy that may bring a better result.

Often, the thing that is causing us frustration is not knowing how to solve our problems. As a result, we just flip back to the old, familiar, unsuccessful ways. Having the patience to seek out and implement a better way will go a long way to relieving your stress.

Stress Buster #8: Learn to Say No

Often our stress is due to the fact that we cannot say no. As a result, we accept too much responsibility. Remember that the world won't end if you don't accept every request that comes your way.

Many people find it difficult to be assertive in certain situations and with certain people. But when you are able to, you can completely avoid many potentially stressful situations. When we don't clearly state our opinion, we can end up in an anxious position. Psychiatrists refer to this as 'suppression' and it can result in low self-esteem and severe depression.

To effectively use this skill, you need to be able to:

- Know when saying no is appropriate (whenever you have a choice)
- Understand the difference between being assertive, being non-assertive and being aggressive
- Practice saying no in simple, non-threatening situations initially before moving on to more challenging situations.

Stress Buster #9: Accept the Unchangeable

When we learn to make a distinction between the changeable and the unchangeable, we can come to peace with the fact that we cannot always be in control. The things we cannot change we should accept. It is encapsulated in what has come to be known as the Serenity Prayer:

> *Grant me the serenity to accept the things I cannot change,*
> *The courage to change the things I can,*
> *And the wisdom to know the difference.*

The key message here is to make things better when you can and to also understand the times when you don't have the power to change a situation. And if you can't change it, it is illogical to stress out about it. Accept it and move on.

If you are stuck in traffic and are late for an appointment, accepting the unchangeable will allow you to be at peace with the situation. Rather than stressing out, you will simply accept the fact that you will be late, turn on the radio and enjoy the music.

Stress Buster #10: Exercise

You know that exercise is a great way to relieve stress. You've probably even heard of the feel-good hormones known as endorphins which lift your mood and generally make you feel good about life.

Regular exercise buys into many of the stress busters that we have already considered. It allows you to carve out of the time of the day that is just for you and also the time when you are able to work on maintaining and improving yourself. This allows you to slow down, build your self-esteem and develop your appreciation for yourself. Studies show that regular cardiovascular exercise significantly improves mental alertness and concentration, reduces stress and improves overall physical and mental wellbeing

The key to exercise success is regularity. Find an activity that you genuinely enjoy and perform it an average of thirty minutes per day. Doing so will enable you to improve your fitness level and lose weight as you get a handle on your stress level.

SUMMARY

Stress is an unavoidable part of all of our lives, but recent research indicates that it affects people aged between 40-54 more than any other age group. A raft of research has shown that stress has a direct impact on our physical health, especially digestion and gut health. The best nutrients to reduce stress are:

- Potassium
- B Vitamins
- Calcium
- Omega-3 Fatty Acids
- Iodine

Reducing your sugar intake will significantly reduce your stress levels. One way you can do this is to switch from a carb-based to a protein-based breakfast. You should also increase your concentration of foods that contain tryptophan as well as those that control your cortisol levels.

Here are 10 foods to include in your diet to help reduce your stress levels:

- Spinach
- Cold water fish
- Swiss Chard
- Cheese
- Plain Yogurt
- Eggs

- Dark Chocolate
- Citrus Fruits
- Walnuts
- Pumpkin seeds

Here are 10 things you can do to keep your stress levels at bay:

- Practice deep nasal breathing
- Learn to appreciate what you have
- Slow down
- Relax your muscles
- Visualize success
- Appreciate yourself
- Change behaviors
- Learn to say no
- Accept the unchangeable
- Exercise

4

WHY DIETS DON'T WORK FOR MOST PEOPLE

"Guilt has no place when it comes to eating"

— EVELYN TRIBOLE

Losing weight is big business. The diet industry is booming with the old standbys like Jenny Craig and Weight Watchers going from strength to strength even as new diets seem to emerge every other day. The integration of diet culture with the social media obsession on physical appearance has fueled the weight loss obsession even further. As a result, many people are still falling into the diet trap despite the overwhelming evidence that diets don't work for most people.

In this chapter, we get to the truth about dieting. You'll discover what really happens to your body when you go on – and off – a diet, how it affects not only your body composition but your overall long-term health, and why diets will never lead to long-term weight loss success. You will also realize that if you've tried and failed on diets in the past, it's not your fault – it's simply further proof that the diet model is fundamentally flawed.

First though, let's consider why diets are still so wildly popular, despite the undeniable evidence that they don't really work.

Why Are Diets So Popular

According to the US Federal Trade Commission, the Diet Industry is the only profitable industry in the world with a 98% failure rate. Think about that for a moment – for every hundred people who go on a diet, only two of them achieve their goal, which is long-term weight loss. Imagine if you were selling a product that failed 98 percent of users. You'd soon be out of business. Yet, the diet industry just keeps going from strength to strength!

How can this be?

A big part of the answer lies in our society's obsession with the thin body. Even in these 'woke' times, Western culture continues to hold up the fat-free body as the physical ideal. It's interesting to note that this is not the case in other parts of the world. Many African tribes, for example, consider excess body fat, especially in females, to be an attractive quality. Not only is it seen as sexy, but it is also an indicator of wealth and status.

In the western world, just the opposite view pervades. Fat is the enemy. And dieting remains the most popular way to defeat it. Here are the top five reasons why we continue to fall into the diet trap.

Diets are Sold as the Solution to Our Problems

The power of the media to influence is stronger than most people realize. From our formative years, we are bombarded with images and messages convincing us that we need to torch fat from our bodies. As a result, many of us link the loss of fat with the achievement of our goals. We tell ourselves that we'll be able to advance in our career when we achieve our goal weight or that we'll be able to start dating online when we get rid of 20 pounds. This provides a very powerful emotional driver to do whatever we have to get the weight off. And when our emotions take over, any intellectual knowledge that dieting isn't going to provide the solution we're looking for will get squashed and we'll allow ourselves to be overtaken by the next and latest glamour fad diet.

The Short-Term Fix Effect

When people do lose weight on a diet, they are celebrated as having achieved something really wonderful. They post before and after pics on Instagram, people comment on their new look and they feel great about themselves. All of that is great. The problem is that 98 percent of people will not only put the weight back on but actually end up heavier than they were before they started the diet.

In effect, going on a diet is a bit like getting a short-term high only to suffer a long-term crash. Even if you know the crash is coming, the lure of the high is very hard to resist!

The Personal Challenge Effect

We all love a challenge. And the diet industry presents us with the opportunity to rely on our willpower and discipline to challenge ourselves in order to conquer our bodies. When people go on diets, they love to talk about it with their peers. Often, they pair up with a friend and it becomes part of a social bonding process. Social media is used as a platform to provide support and reinforcement. The diet, in effect, is part of the relationship.

Diet challenges are especially attractive. These are increasingly being pushed online with the social aspect and the prospect of winning and becoming a social media' star' drawing in many people.

Diets Put You on Auto-Pilot

Diets provide a paint-by-numbers approach to weight loss. So long as we buy the book or sign up to the program, we don't have to think about what we should eat and when. We simply follow the template. Many people find that to be an extremely attractive proposition.

Celebrity Endorsements

Celebrities have been making money from diet endorsements for a long time. They continue to do so because their endorsements carry a lot of weight (no pun intended). Social media platforms have allowed celebrities to share more of their lives with their fans than ever. As a result, we get to see them following a diet as they go through their normal routine. Of course, they are really nothing more than the social media equivalent of product placement ads but they can make a big impression on someone who idolizes that celebrity.

WHY DIETS DON'T WORK

So far in this chapter, I've made it clear that diets are not the solution if you are after long-term weight loss. Let's now back up that assertion. Here are a half dozen reasons why you should never go on a diet.

Your Metabolism is Negatively Affected

Most people throw around the word metabolism without really knowing what it is. We've been conditioned to thinking that we've either got a fast or slow metabolism, with most of us convincing ourselves that we've got an extremely slow one – otherwise, we'd be able to lose weight, right?

The truth is that your metabolism – the rate at which all of the chemical reactions that occur within your body in order to keep you alive – is constantly fluctuating.

The metabolism was created to deal with the conditions that our original ancestors faced. Back then, finding food took a great deal of energy. In fact, it was likely that a person would go for a lengthy period of time without any food at all. The metabolism was designed in such a way that, when we ate less, it slowed down. This was a natural starvation response to preserve calories so that we had enough energy to carry us through.

Today, of course, we hardly ever find ourselves in a real life or death starvation situation. Yet, the metabolism works the same as it did back then. When we *choose* to eat less, such as when we go on a restricted-calorie diet, the metabolism will gradually slow down. That means that we will be burning energy more slowly.

As a result of this natural 'starvation response' the body actually works against dieting. It is doing so in order to prepare you for a coming famine, with the effect that you will actually store fat more readily. Your body doesn't know that you are consciously choosing to cut back on calories. It responds as if you were in an emergency situation to prevent you from starving. Hormonal changes take place to allow you to hoard body fat as stored energy just the same way a bear does in preparation for hibernation over the winter.

Psychological Defeatism

When we go on a diet, we become obsessed with food. It's the classic pink elephant scenario. If you are told not to think about a pink elephant, what will constantly pop into your head over the next five minutes?

You got it . . . images of pink elephants!

Same thing with food. If you are told not to eat certain foods for a long period of time, you will particularly think about the foods that have been forbidden to you. This makes the task of sticking to the diet that much harder.

Another thing that happens when we restrict our eating is that we get more stressed. A 2010 study out of Los Angeles proved for the first time that diets are stressful and lead to the release of the cortisol hormone. This, in turn, leads to the temptation to binge eat and keeps you awake at night, inhibiting the release of the hunger or satiety hormones ghrelin and leptin. In these ways, the stress will also make you fatter.

Research shows that the brain responds differently to food when you are dieting. It becomes far more tuned in to food. As a result, you will pick up flavors and aromas more readily. When you come in contact with appetizing food, your taste buds will salivate faster than when you are not dieting. It has even been shown that the prefrontal cortex, which is the portion of the brain that controls temptation, is less active when you are dieting.

Weight Loss Obsession

A major problem with low-calorie diets is that they do not differentiate between weight loss and fat loss. You should never be interested in losing pure weight. Being obsessed with bringing your weight down on the scale is misguided – pure and simple.

The bathroom scale cannot differentiate between muscle and fat. Nor can it tell if you are losing water or vital minerals. All it can tell you is that your overall body weight has gone down. That, in itself, is a useless piece of information.

You never want to lose muscle. Yet, on most calorie-restricted diets, that is exactly what you are losing. Muscle weighs five times more than fat. So, when a person's body goes into starvation response because they have severely cut back their caloric intake, the body turns to its muscle stores and starts to catabolize itself.

When you step on the scale, you feel elated. The scale has come down. But what have you actually done to your body? You have robbed it of its body shaping, firming, strength-enhancing muscle mass. Meanwhile, most of your fat is still there, where it's always been.

You can be on a calorie-reduced diet and still be incredibly unhealthy. Likewise, you can actually increase your calories by eating more nutritionally rich food whilst exercising regularly and you can actually lose fat and gain muscle. Just think how much food professional athletes put away on a daily basis. In 2014, Olympic wrestling gold medal winner Kurt Angle revealed that he would have around 7 meals per day, eating every two hours. He was of course, on an elite training regime, but he was in incredible shape and far from being considered fat.

Reduced calorie diets will also squeeze water weight from your body, especially in the initial stages. We've already discussed the vital importance of water in the body, so you know that is not a good thing. Yet, again, it fools people into thinking that they are losing body fat.

Research Show It Doesn't Work for Most of Us

The conventional wisdom about losing weight hasn't changed for more than a hundred years. That thinking tells us that it is all about calories. If you consume calories in excess of those burned through metabolism and inactivity, you'll get fat. So, obviously, in order to lose that fat, you've got to eat fewer calories and exercise more.

The only problem is that millions of people have been doing just that – and actually getting fatter! There is also a mountain of both anecdotal and research-based evidence to show that this approach needs to not be looked at so simplistically. Let's take a look at an example of a calorie-reduced diet.

In one study published in the journal *Lancet* in 2009, participants with an average age of 36 and an average Body Mass Index (BMI) of 35 were put on a calorie-reduced diet (1,000 calories reduction) for a full 12 months. Half of them also exercised. After twelve months, the results were as follows:

Diet only group: 0.9 kg lost
Diet and exercise: 2.2 kg lost

Another 12-month study involved people with an average age of 42 who had an average BMI of 36.5. These people were put on a diet of between 1,200 and 1,500 calories per day. Half of them also did regular aerobic exercise, resistance exercise. Results were:

Diet only group: 4.6 kg lost
Diet and exercise: 5.2 kg lost

A third study had people with an average age of 45 and an average BMI of 36 put on a low-fat diet containing 800-1,000 calories per day. Again, half of them were given exercise in the form of brisk walking for 3 miles, 5 times per week. This lasted for two years. Results were:

Diet only group: 2.1 kg lost
Diet and exercise: 2.5 kg lost

Our final study involved men with an average age of 43 and an average BMI of 25.5. They followed a low-fat, high-carb diet for 12 months. Once more, some of the group added exercise, this time in the form of 30 minutes of aerobic exercise, 4-5 times per week. Results were:

Diet only group: No change in weight
Diet and exercise: 1.9 kg lost

Let's now take a look at a summary of those results . . .

Study	Length (months)	Weight change (kg) – diet only	Weight change (kg) – diet and exercise
1	12	-0.9	-2.2
2	12	-4.6	-5.2
3	24	-2.1	-2.5
4	12	0.0	-1.9
Average	-	-1.9	-2.95

So, what do we learn from these diet studies?

After an average of 12 months of hardcore dieting, the average weight loss was just 2 kg. Even when exercise was added to the equation, the average weight loss only went up to 3 kg. Keep in mind, too, that the people on these studies had an abundance of professional support and guidance. The bottom line is that traditional dieting methods, those based on caloric restriction, are in many cases, a fast track to failure.

FAD DIET DANGER SIGNS

From what we've considered so far in this chapter, it should be clear that fad diets are just another bad food habit that needs to be avoided. So, let's pause for a moment and consider just what a fad diet is.

The word diet has had its original meaning corrupted over the past 100 years. Originally your diet simply referred to what you ate. But now the word is used to describe a period of restricted eating where you cut back on calories and avoid certain types of food. A fad diet will often center around a specific type of food. Others severely restrict or cut out a food group like carbohydrates.

Here are the characteristics of a fad diet to look out for and avoid . . .

- The diet cuts out a macronutrient – any type of diet that severely restricts one of the food groups is bad news. Not only is it extremely difficult to sustain such a diet, but you will struggle to meet your body's fuel needs if you cut back too much on any macronutrient.
- They describe their diet as being 'easy' – losing weight the right way isn't easy. With all of the bad food choices that we are surrounded with, it requires consistency, discipline and self-control. Any diet that tells you otherwise is lying to you.
- The diet promises rapid weight loss – you can lose weight fast but you cannot lose fat fast. Slow and steady fat loss is the way to go.
- The diet requires that you follow strict rules that are unrealistic in the real world.
- The diet claims scientific backing but it is based on in-house research or anecdotal evidence.

Negative Effects of Fad Diets

Fads are not only ineffective. They can also be dangerous. Here are 10 negative effects that may result from going on a fad diet...

- Dehydration
- Overhydration
- Muscle loss
- Reduced bone density
- Lack of energy
- Headaches
- Low blood sugar
- Heart damage
- Nutritional deficiencies
- Constipation

What Happens When the Diet Ends?

By its definition, a fad diet comes to an end. So, what happens when that expiration date rolls around? For many dieters, the end of the diet is binge time. They compensate for all those weeks of restrictive eating by splurging out on the sugary, sweet foods they've been missing on. This binge eating is not just the result of a lack of willpower; the diet model itself actually drives it.

Diets create forbidden foods in the mind of the dieter. As we noted with the example of pink elephants, we can't help but obsess over these out-of-bounds foods. The brain is overstimulated to light up when these foods come on our radar. It's hardly surprising that when the diet is over and the restrictions are off, we go crazy and splurge on cakes, cookies and junk food.

When a dieter goes on a post-diet binge, they'll often justify it by telling themselves that it is a one-off – and that they deserve it. But it is hardly ever a one-off! In fact, it is part of a vicious cycle. Binge eating leads to shame and guilt, which causes one to jump onto another fad diet. When they come off the diet, they binge again and the process repeats. This cycle has been the pattern for millions of people for years.

WHAT ABOUT INTERMITTENT FASTING?

One of the most popular diets to emerge in recent years has been Intermittent Fasting. It is centered more around the timing of your eating than the actual foods that you eat. Intermittent fasting involves periods of fasting followed by an eating window. The fasting period could range from 12 hours to more than 40 hours. The most popular form of IF is the 16:8 diet, in which the dieter fasts for 16 hours of each 24-hour period and eats for the remaining 8 hours. Here is how it may look . . .

You stop eating at 7pm. You then fast until 11am the following morning. Then, between 11am and 7pm you eat your food.

So, how effective is Intermittent Fasting when it comes to long-term fat loss? A recent major study suggests that there is no evidence that time-restricted eating works as a weight-loss strategy. In the study, one group of people were put on an IF regimen of 8 hour feeding windows and 16 hour fasting periods each day. At the end of 12 weeks, they had lost an average of 2 pounds. Another group ate normally with similar foods at the same caloric intake for 12 weeks. They lost an average of 1.5 pounds. The researchers concluded that the difference was not statistically significant. The fasting group were also shown to lose more muscle mass over the period of the study than the control group.

There does, however, need to be more research on the effects of intermittent fasting for long-term weight loss. The research that currently exists, however, suggests that it may not be the panacea that many are proclaiming it to be.

SUMMARY

In this chapter, we have clearly established that dieting is not the solution to long-term weight loss. Despite having a 98 percent failure rate, however, they continue to be the weight loss option of choice for the majority of people as a result of . . .

- Media influence
- The short-term fix effect
- The solution to all our problems effect
- Their paint by numbers approach
- Celebrity endorsements

Yet, despite how popular fad diets are, the science of how the body works means that they can never be successful. When you go on a diet the following things occur . . .

- Your metabolism slows down
- Your body kicks into fight or flight mode
- Your cortisol levels increase
- Stress levels rise
- You fixate on forbidden foods
- You tend to lose muscle tissue, water and minerals over fat

Then when you go off the diet, there is a high likelihood that you will binge eat, which leads to rebound weight gain. In fact, research confirms that the vast majority of dieters end up fatter in the long run than before they started the diet.

The message is clear – if you are interested in long-term fat loss, steer clear of diets!

STEP TWO. CHANGING MINDSET

5

IDENTIFYING THE RULES & HABITS WE NOW LIVE BY

"You don't have to see the whole staircase, just take the first step"

— MARTIN LUTHER KING

In the first section of this book, we have established that our eating habits are heavily influenced by our upbringing and our environment. But that doesn't mean that our nutritional future is predetermined. We all have the power within us to break free of the bad nutritional habits that have got us to where we are. The first step in that process is to identify the habits that have developed as subconscious eating rules in our own lives. By becoming mindful of what we are doing, we will be in a position to challenge and change it.

Want an example of how powerful mindfulness is when it comes to our eating habits? Like most people, you may have the habit of chowing down on potato chips while watching TV. But try eating a packet of potato chips while you're staring at your naked self in the mirror or, better yet, standing on the bathroom scales! Suddenly those chips won't be so appetizing. What's the difference? You're now mindfully aware of the consequences of your eating habit!

In this chapter, I'm going to challenge you to identify the eating habits that have become ingrained in your life over the years. To do this, you'll be presented with a number of interactive activities that will help you to become a mindful detective about your current eating habits.

To successfully identify and then overcome your unproductive eating habits, you need to go into this process without judgment. Now is not the time to condemn yourself or feel guilty about the bad eating habits you have developed. Rather than being judgmental, be curious. Curiosity opens you up to creativity, which is the spark that leads to positive change.

MINDFUL EATING

Most people go through life on automatic pilot. They perform their daily activities without any thought while their brain is consumed with something else. As a result, they miss the gift of the present while their mind is either regretting the past or worrying about the future. Mindfulness is the counter to living your life on automatic pilot. Although it is a relatively new concept in the consciousness of the western world, mindfulness has been around for a long time. In the 1960s, the famous missionary Mother Teresa summed up the whole essence of mindfulness with this simple statement...

> "Be happy in the moment. That's enough. Each moment is all we need, not more."

The opposite of mindfulness is mindlessness. It involves doing what you have always done without thinking about it. When you live like that, you are not in control of your life. Mindfulness puts you back in the driver's seat, allowing you to live a purposeful life.

Here are 8 principles that form the basis of mindfulness:

- Be in the moment, slow down and think about what you are doing NOW
- Realize that you have the power to change
- Trust your gut instincts
- Attune your mind and body
- Become aware of your habits
- Be curious, not judgmental
- Take responsibility for your actions
- Maintain an open, flexible mind

Mindful eating applies the principles of mindfulness to your eating habits. It is all about being fully aware of your habits, cravings and behaviors regarding the nutrients that go into your body. When you eat mindfully, you are able to eat the foods that you want when you want to rather than being a slave to your habitual behaviors.

Many people find that mindful eating becomes a catalyst to taking control of other areas of their lives as well. As a result, they become more empowered, more connected and happier.

Here is a 6-step process that will help you to become a mindful eater . . .

Control What Comes into the House

Mindful eating begins at the supermarket. That is the source of most of the food that comes into your house. Start at the vegetable section and spend time exploring. Choose a wide range of vegetable types and colors. Look for veggies that are new to you and give them a try.

Shop on the outskirts of the store. Think about the nutritional impact of everything that goes into your trolley. If you allow yourself a treat food, do it mindfully, having planned it into your week. Be especially in the moment when you are at the checkout as that is where the most tempting sugar-laden snacks will be hanging out.

Don't Allow Yourself to Get Too Hungry

If you come to the dinner table with a ravenous appetite, there is a very high likelihood that you will stuff yourself so full of food that you'll end up feeling very uncomfortable. You won't be thinking about what you're eating or about your satiety cues.

You can avoid getting overly hungry between meals by eating a quality source of lean protein with each meal, spacing your meals about three hours apart and drinking plenty of water throughout the day.

Buy Smaller Plates

The diameter of the average dinner plate sold over the past 60 years has expanded right along with people's waistlines. In the 1950's that diameter was 9 inches, while today it is 13.5 inches. Most of us have been conditioned to cleaning up everything on our plate, even if we feel we've had enough. This leads to overeating and a daily caloric surplus, which leads to fat storage.

The simple remedy is to buy smaller dinner plates. Reduce down to 9 inches and your waistline will also come down.

Savor Your Food

Before you even take your first bite, consciously look over the plate and take it all in. Think about how those different flavors are going to entice your taste buds and about how the nutrients contained in the foods on your plate are going to make your body better. Take a moment to appreciate the effort that went into preparing the food and, if you are religious, thank the Creator for being the ultimate source of it.

Engage All of Your Senses

When that food heads your way, engage all of your senses in order to fully appreciate it. Take in the aroma, colors and texture. And then, when you put it in your mouth, see if you can identify all of the ingredients, including the sauces and seasonings.

Chew Your Food Thoroughly

Chewing your food well will help you to slow down in your eating. It will also maximize the release of digestive enzymes in the mouth. In addition, the more thoroughly you chew your food the less work your digestive system will have to do. And, according to recent research, the more you chew, the more satisfied you will be with your meal and the fewer overall calories you will consume.

Researchers have made links between chewing and enhanced cognitive benefits. Neural circuits in the brain connect the act of chewing with the hippocampus, which controls cognitive functioning. Chewing has also been shown to have a positive correlation with attention and focus.

Chew each bite a minimum of 10 times before swallowing it down.

SLOWING DOWN: THE ESSENCE OF MINDFUL EATING

A habit that many people have developed over their life's course is to shovel food into their mouth, one spoonful after the other, without a break. It's as if they're in a race to see who can finish eating first. Generally, these people tend to have too much fat on their bodies, whereas skinnier people will tend to eat more slowly. Let's find out why.

You get fuller faster when you eat slower. This is because your brain gets a chance to say "I'm full" at a faster rate, as opposed to just shoveling the food in and ending up with a stomach ache. For us to feel full, the brain needs to receive signals from hormones located in the gastrointestinal tract. This hormonal signaling system is a complex process by which leptin and cholecystokinin (CCK) amplify the feeling of fullness. It takes a full twenty minutes, however, for the brain to get the signal that you are full. Shoveling the calories into your mouth at a rate of knots is going to massively oversupply your food needs. You will end up wearing the excess around your waist.

When we eat properly – i.e., slowly – the hormone leptin interacts with the neurotransmitter dopamine to produce a sensation of pleasure. When we eat too fast, however, dopamine is not released. We derive neither a feeling of fullness nor pleasure. This leads us to keep on eating.

Your stomach does not have teeth. So, everything that you put into it has to be broken down. When you eat fast, your body doesn't have a chance to process the food. As you chew it in your mouth, saliva begins the digestive process. By the time it goes down your throat, a large part of the digestive process has already been accomplished. But, when you simply swallow it down without chewing, you are placing undue stress on your gut. As a result, large pieces of unprocessed food can become trapped in the stomach, leading to gastric discomfort.

Eating too quickly can also lead to bloating. This problem occurs when too much air enters the digestive tract, as often happens when you eat too fast.

People who eat too fast tend not to enjoy their food as much. Food is one of the great pleasures in life. It deserves to be treated with respect, to be savored, relished and lingered over. Those who eat to complete are missing out on so much. They are depriving themselves of the exquisite joy of flavor.

In addition to the pleasure of enjoying your food, slowing down your eating allows you to enjoy one of the other great joys of eating – socialization. Sharing a meal is perhaps the most universally accepted and widely enjoyed means of sharing time with others. In this regard, we can take a lesson from the Mediterranean world.

For centuries, the inhabitants of the 16 countries surrounding the Mediterranean have been experiencing a unique level of health, longevity and weight control. More and more people around the world have been joining them, not just to achieve optimum health but to shed excess body fat. The biggest difference between the way they eat and the way the Western world eats is that they take more time to enjoy and savor their meals.

ACTION PLAN

Eating slowly will take effort. In fact, it will require what has come to be known as mindful eating on your part. Mindful eating simply involves being consciously in the moment when you are eating. Here are four practical steps to help you to develop mindful eating and thus slow down and enjoy your food.

Step One

Plan to spend 30 minutes eating your larger meals. Get out of the mindset of dinner being an inconvenience that you have to get out of the way in order to get back to the TV set. Try to have the whole family sitting at the dinner table, turn off the TV (and your phone), and initiate a discussion. If your family isn't used to this, it may seem a little strange at first. You can help by having a strategy – ask each family member for their highlight (or lowlight) of the day.

Step Two

Count to ten before each bite. This will allow you to assess just how hungry you actually are. Think about it. If you're already feeling full, you are allowed to stop. Counting to ten will also provide time for you to fully digest the mouthful that has come before.

Step Three

Talk during your meal – when you're at a social gathering, don't think so much about the food. Think more about the company that you are with. You are eating so you can stay alive – and enjoy the association of your loved ones. Focusing on eating rather than communicating is akin to not seeing the forest for the trees!

Step Four

The body triggers its sensation for food and water based on diminished energy levels. These two sensations reach the brain together – and most people interpret them to be a sensation just to eat. The body does not send a separate signal for thirst and another one for food. As a result, we often reach for food when we should be reaching for water.

If we could separate these two sensations, then we would be at an immediate advantage in the battle to control our body fat levels.

Well, we can – and here's how:

> **Drink a glass of water before you eat.**

When you do that, you will satisfy the body's need for hydration and you will prevent yourself from overeating. You should also drink water with your meal.

IDENTIFYING YOUR EATING HABITS

It's time now to take a close look at the eating habits that have developed in your life and that unconsciously dictate the way that you fuel your body. Not all of your eating habits will be detrimental. Some of them will be positive and you will definitely want to retain them. Others, however, will be clearly bad for you and you will be far better off without them. The first step to ditching them is identifying what they are.

7-Day Food Diary

In order to bring your unconscious eating habits to the forefront of your mind, you will have to do a little detective work. It begins with a food diary. Over the next 7 days, I want you to keep a diary of everything you eat.

You can either use a notebook as your food diary or download a food journal app. Here are the things you should make a record of:

- Date
- Time
- Place (e.g. at home in front of TV)
- Food item and quantity
- How you felt before and after eating
- Your hunger level before and after

6 Food Diary Tips

Record Everything

If it travels between your lips, it needs to be recorded in your food diary. That includes everything you drink as well as what you eat. Don't dismiss those nibbly snacks you eat on the run or even the sneaky mouthfuls you gulp down when cooking - record it all!

Break food meals down into ingredients. So, rather than writing 'chicken sandwich', take note of how many pieces of bread you had, how much chicken and what, if any, sauces or other condiments you included.

Record your water intake as well.

Record Accurate Quantities

You should measure out the quantities of foods that you're eating with a pair of kitchen scales, along with measuring cups and bowls. The more accurate you are in recording your food intake, the easier it will be to analyze your habits once you're done.

Accurate Time and Place

Be as specific as you can in recording the time that you eat. So, rather than writing down 'afternoon snack,' jot down the actual time. This will help you to more accurately identify your eating patterns.

You also need to record where you eat in the home. Was it in front of the TV or at the dinner table, in bed, or at the kitchen aisle?

Emotional State

Were you feeling stressed immediately before eating? Was food your comfort? After the meal, did you actually feel comfort, or was guilt the overriding emotion? Whatever it was, write it all down.

Physical Reactions

Did you experience gas or bloating after the meal? Be sure to record all of your physical reactions to the food you eat.

Use the Hunger Gauge to Record your Hunger Level

The Hunger Gauge was created by nutritionists to help their clients train themselves to eat as a response to feeling hungry rather than as a result of social or other cues.

The hunger gauge has the following 6 levels to follow:

1. You are desperately hungry and experiencing clear physical signs of hunger, such as feeling shaky or faint.
2. You are very hungry; your stomach is rumbling and you feel a little tired.
3. You are moderately hungry; you have an appetite for food and a pleasant sense of anticipation.
4. You feel satisfied. You could perhaps be tempted to eat dessert, but it is not essential.
5. You are too full; you left it a little late to stop eating because you couldn't resist the temptation of another small helping.
6. You are very full; you ignored all the signs to stop eating and now feel weighed down. You may also experience indigestion and heartburn.

Note down a before and after Hunger Gauge rating for every meal that you record in your food diary.

Listing Your Eating Habits

Once you have completed 7 days of your food diary, you will have a key resource to help you identify your eating habits. Take a piece of paper (or create a document on your device) and divide it into two columns. On the left-hand side, you will list all of the bad eating habits that are part of your life. On the right-hand side, note down all of the good nutrition habits that you have developed.

Here is an example of the common good and bad habits that ingrain themselves as the rules of eating for many people...

Bad Eating Habits	Good Eating Habits
o Eating in front of TV o Eating too fast o Eating for comfort o Eating ready meals o Eating out too often o Hangovers and eating junk food o Fasting then binge eating o Weighing yourself too much o Going shopping hungry o Going back for seconds o Serving food at the table which makes getting seconds easier o Rewarding your good eating with desert too often o Snacking while cooking o Taking too long between meals o Portion sizes o Fixating on the bathroom scales o Takeaways o Weeks off, weekends on o The ' I've been good" rule	o Snacking on fruit o Eating frequent small meals o Eating slowly o Limiting red meat o Drinking water with meals

ANALYZE YOUR EATING TRIGGERS

Breaking the link between your emotional state and your food intake can be the first step to successful weight control. Recognizing that there is an emotional dimension to your eating will help you adopt healthy eating habits.

Having completed your food diary and listed your habits, you are in a great position to analyze both to identify your emotional eating triggers. Use your food diary to answer the following questions:

	YES	NO
Do you eat more when you are alone, such as when watching TV?		
Do you give yourself 'rewards' of chocolate or sweets if you have had a difficult day?		
If you have broken your diet and eaten a rich dessert, do you feel so upset that you might as well give up and eat what you like for the rest of the day?		
Does looking in the mirror or weighing yourself make you so depressed that you need a treat to cheer yourself up?		
Do you eat high fat energy foods, such as chips and chocolate to give you a pick-me-up boost when you are down?		

The Most Common Emotional Eating Triggers

Analyze your food diary in relation to these 6 most common emotional eating triggers:

Stress

When we get stressed, the body overproduces the hormone cortisol. Cortisol triggers a desire for salty, sweet and fried foods that deliver a quick energy boost. When under stress, we use food as a numbing strategy to distract us from the problem weighing on our minds. Research also shows that eating sugary foods can actually stimulate the pleasure centers in the brain in a similar way to such drugs like cocaine or heroin. Dopamine, the feel-good hormone, surges into the brain's pleasure center at the same time that endogenous opioids, the brain's natural painkillers, induce more positive feelings.

To identify if you are a stress eater, go back to your food diary and take a look at your Hunger Gauge numbers and your emotional state when eating various meals. If you can pinpoint several times during the week when you reached for sugar-laden foods at times when your hunger gauge was low and your emotional state was heightened, then you are a stress eater.

Burying Your Emotions

Can you identify periods during the week when you ate in order to bury disturbing emotions or memories? That piece of cake and cup of coffee becomes a soothing mechanism that allows us to put a band-aid over the troubling emotions that are gnawing away deep inside. You are, in effect, self-medicating with food. Meanwhile, the root emotional problem is festering - and you're gaining weight!

Boredom

Were there times during the week that you were doing something that you just couldn't get your mind excited about and then, as if on autopilot, you found yourself wandering to the fridge and opening the door in search of a snack? This is boredom eating. Boredom generates feelings of negativity, lack of fulfillment and frustration. Our natural reaction to those feelings is to find ways to reverse them. Food can easily become the trigger to doing so.

The thought of satisfying our taste buds with a delicious treat can be the counter to the negativity that boredom produces. Of course, that awesome taste is only momentary, so we eat more and more to keep feeling those positive emotions. But then what happens? Usually, we are plagued by feelings of disgust or guilt at our lack of self-control. And the boredom remains!

Social Influences

Food is the lubrication of social interaction. When we have visitors, or when we are visiting others, we often feel a social obligation to serve or bring an item of food. We eat it because it is served to us, not because we are hungry. Many people also eat out of nervousness when they are with others. Look back through your food diary to see if you can identify situations where you ate in social situations when your Hunger Gauge was higher than 3.

Binge Eating Disorder

Binge eating disorder, although not as prominently discussed as bulimia and anorexia nervosa, is actually the most common eating disorder in both the United States and the United Kingdom. In fact, binge eating disorder is three times more common in the United States than anorexia and bulimia combined.

Binge eating disorder is recognized by the Diagnostic and Statistical Manual of Mental Disorders (DSM-V), a standard classification used by health professionals, as a mental disorder. According to the DSM-V, binge eating disorder has the following characteristics:

- Recurring episodes of eating large amounts of food rapidly to the point of discomfort.
- During the eating, the person feels a sense of loss of control, as if they can't stop until there is no food left.
- Eating an amount of food that is significantly

more than most would eat in similar circumstances in a short amount of time.
- Loss of control over how much/what one is eating, feeling like one cannot stop eating.
- Episodes of binge eating also must include at least three of the following characteristics: Eating rapidly and to the point of discomfort. Eating when one is not physically hungry. Eating alone so others do not know how much one is eating.
- Episodes followed by feelings of shame, guilt, disgust Distress around the binge-eating behavior.

Unlike other eating disorders such as bulimia nervosa, there are no compensatory activities involved, such as purging, taking laxatives, or excessive amounts of exercise. Binge eating has been described as a tornado that sweeps in and overtakes a person. When the urge to binge strikes, they feel unable to do anything about it. In a sense, the person is a bystander in their own body; all they can do is to watch themselves, as if from a distance, as they perpetuate the same desperate behavior time and again.

Binge eating is distinct from occasional overeating. It is accompanied by a complete loss of physical self-control where the person cannot possibly stop eating despite the physical discomfort that they feel.

There is no one identifiable cause of binge eating disorder. It results from a perfect storm aligning a number of contributing factors. These are a combination of genetic and environmental factors. With regard to the interplay between genetics and environment, Dr. Francis Collins of the US National Institute of Health commented, "genetics loads the gun; environment pulls the trigger."

The following factors work together to contribute to the development of the disorder:

- Genetic factors - recent research has pinpointed a gene that may be a genetic risk factor for binge eating. This gene is called cytoplasmic FMR1-interacting protein 2 (CY- FIP2).
- Hormonal irregularities - sufferers of binge eating disorders have been shown to have increased levels of the hunger-inducing hormone ghrelin.
- Receiving the message from parents and others that food is a comfort and soothing mechanism.
- Being raised in an environment where there is a constant focus on dieting and weight loss.
- Life stressors that arise during teen years such as leaving home, relationship problems, academic pressures and other unfamiliar, challenging situations.
- Life transitions such as relationship breakup, moving to a new city or losing one's job.
- Depression or anxiety.
- Perfectionist tendencies.
- Addictive personality traits.

BREAKING FREE FROM BINGE EATING

Millions of people have managed to break the shackles of binge eating and so can you. Here are seven proven strategies that you can employ to overcome this condition:

Journaling

Journaling can be used as a therapeutic tool to help you when you get the urge to binge eat. Even though it will be difficult, rather than going with the surge of desire to begin eating, stop, breathe, count to 10 and reach for your journal. Now explore on paper the emotions that are driving your binge desire. Is it boredom? Loneliness? A painful memory or experience? Will food really be the panacea to this problem that your emotional driver is telling you that it will be?

When you write openly and honestly about your emotions, you will be forcing yourself to confront your emotions rather than running away from them.

Alternative Activities

By having an alternative coping mechanism in place prior to the binge urge overtaking you, you will be far more likely to resist it and not give in to the temptation. Your alternative activity could be to go for a walk, contact a support person, listen to your favorite music, exercise, take a bubble bath or practice a mindful breathing exercise.

Don't Skip Meals

It has been shown that planning out regular meal times and sticking to them is one of the proven ways to lessen the occurrence of binge eating. Plan your meals every three hours apart and stick to that schedule.

Practice Mindfulness

A meta-study that analyzed 14 studies found that the regular practice of mindfulness significantly decreased the incidence of binge eating. We have already discussed how mindful eating practices can help you to break free from bad eating habits. When it comes to binge eating, the key skill to develop is an awareness of your actual physical hunger level. Go back to the Hunger Gauge and rate yourself. If your rating is 4 or higher, forbid yourself from eating!

Drink Plenty of Water

Staying well hydrated will keep you feeling full throughout the day which will, in turn, make you less inclined to develop the binge eating urge. Drinking water before a meal will also make you less likely to binge. In one study, it was shown that consuming 500 mls of water before one meal per day decreased total daily caloric consumption by 13 percent in comparison to a control group.

Increase Fiber Consumption

Fiber is a great way to keep yourself full. That is because it adds bulk to your diet without adding extra calories. Not only will it help you to feel full sooner, but because it takes longer than other foods to move through your system, it will keep you full longer.

When fiber fills up your stomach, it stimulates receptors that send messages to your brain that tell you to stop eating.

Soluble fiber decreases enterohepatic recycling of bile acids which can decrease serum cholesterol levels. Insoluble fiber will add bulk to stools while also decreasing colon cancer risk.

An added benefit of soluble fiber is that, when it absorbs water, it forms a gel in the lower intestine. This slows the absorption of blood sugar. This, in turn, leads to lower insulin levels, which makes you less likely to store body fat.

Here's how you will benefit from these adaptations:

- Increased satiety
- Lowered blood fat and cholesterol
- Reduced risk of colon cancer
- Proper intestinal motility
- Enhanced gut health

When it comes to fruits and vegetables, the majority of the fiber is found in the skin, membrane and seeds. That's why you need to be eating fruits with the skin on.

If you are a woman, aim for 35 grams per day.
If you are a man, aim for 48 grams per day.

Be sure to drink plenty of water when you eat fiber. You'll need a minimum of eight glasses each day in order to keep the fiber moving through your system. Water, of course, also helps to keep you full.

Increase Protein Intake

Increasing your protein intake will help to fill you up and keep you satisfied throughout the day. The word protein is derived from the Greek *proteios*, meaning 'most important.' Along with carbohydrates and fats, it is one of the three macronutrients. We all know that protein is the key macro or muscle gain. Fewer people realize that it is also the main nutrient for satiety. Therefore, keeping a high protein intake will allow you to feel full all day long, which will make you far less likely to binge eat.

There are three ways that protein helps in this regard:

- It helps us to build lean muscle tissue. Once you take away the water, muscle tissue is almost exclusively made of protein.
- Protein has a higher thermic effect than either carbohydrates or fat. During the process of digestion, some 25% of protein calories are used during digestion, compared to just 6-8% for carbs and 2-3% for fat.

- Protein fills you up, which helps you to go longer between meals without feeling hungry again.

There are a large number of studies that have shown that the combination of these three factors are effective factors in fat loss. People who are assigned to eat more protein lose more fat. Retain more muscle tissue, have less hunger and eat less total food.

In contrast, studies have shown that lower protein intake leads to overeating, fat gain, and muscle loss. Such results have led some researchers to propound the protein leverage hypothesis, which states that humans have the ability to keep track of how much protein we've eaten. This tracking system, it is claimed, is the ultimate controller of appetite. We eat more food when we have less protein in our meals and less when we have more.

According to the protein leverage hypothesis, then, hunger is really a quest for protein.

This protein leverage hypothesis seems to gel with what we see in society. Researchers have been scratching their heads for decades at the statistics which show that the wealthiest people in society are also the leanest, while the poorest people are the fattest. Of the three macronutrients, protein is the most expensive. So, if all that you eat is low-quality, mass-produced food, you'll need a lot more of it to reach your body's internal protein target.

Let's take a look at some of the exciting research that has ramped up protein's fat loss profile in recent years.

- A 2014 study investigated the effects of protein intake on between-meal snacking and resultant weight loss. A group was given dairy protein every four hours as compared to a control group who only ate protein once per day but were also fed every four hours. Not only did the protein group resist the urge to graze between meals, their average weight loss after 28 days was 17% greater than the control group.
- A 2011 study of overweight and obese men by Leidy, et al. revealed that upping your protein intake while reducing carbs at every meal of the day resulted in a greater loss of body fat than only eating protein in the evening.
- In 2011 a study was undertaken that showed that eating an ample amount of protein for breakfast significantly reduced food cravings throughout the remainder of the day. The test subjects were teenagers who normally skipped breakfast. They were exposed to visual food responses after being given a normal versus a high-protein breakfast. Those who were given the high-protein breakfast exhibited significantly greater neural resistance to the temptations shown to them.
- Many studies have shown that eating protein throughout the day preserves lean muscle mass when a person is losing body fat. This was seen in a 2008 study by Bopp, et al. which was published in the "Journal of the American Dietetic Association"
- A 2002 study specifically showed that eating more protein leads to an increase in fat loss.

Another major advantage of protein? Unlike carbohydrates or fats, taking in high levels of protein does not play havoc with your insulin levels!

BREAKING FREE FROM THE BINGE-RESTRICT CYCLE

The binge-restrict cycle is similar to the diet-relapse cycle that we discussed in the previous chapter, just on a more condensed time scale. Here's how it goes . . .

- You binge eat
- You experience feelings of guilt and shame
- You resolve to do better in the future
- You overcompensate by with some form of eating restriction
- You binge eat again

In order to break free from this cycle, you need to focus on the two key factors of physical hunger and negative emotions. After a binge eating episode, you need to resist the temptation to cut back on your next meal. Those feelings of guilt are only natural but realize that you do not have to be stuck into a cycle that perpetuates the problem. Focus on the next meal, which should be around 3 hours after your binge eating episode. This meal will probably be significantly smaller than usual, but it is vital that you have some food, just as you normally would.

You also need to break free from the categorization of food as good or bad. Food is just food. It should not have a moral tag attached to it. When you are able to de-stigmatize certain foods, you no longer view them as temptation foods. Often people binge on these so-called forbidden foods, but when you include them in moderation as part of a blanched eating plan, you take their power to tempt you into an overeating episode.

Another key to breaking out of the binge-restrict cycle is to not be too harsh on yourself. When you begin to experience those feelings of shame, put on the mental brakes. Remind yourself that you are not a robot. You are going to have slip ups, but you are smarter than falling back into the usual cycle.

Getting out of the binge-restrict cycle isn't easy. You probably won't succeed on the first occasion. Achieving long-term success is all about forgiving yourself when you slip up and being patient with yourself.

SUMMARY

In this chapter, you have closely analyzed the way you eat to identify your good and bad habits. You have kept a detailed 7-day food diary and then poured over it in order to bring to the forefront of your mind the unconscious habits that have built up over your lifetime to produce your personal rules of eating. We have also examined some of the more frequent habits that people create for themselves, both consciously and unconsciously.

We've discovered in this chapter that a powerful impetus to breaking free from the eating rules that enslave us is the concept of mindfulness. Mindful eating involves:

- Controlling what comes into the house
- Not allowing yourself to get too hungry
- Buying smaller plates
- Savoring your food
- Engaging all your senses
- Chewing your food thoroughly
- Slowing down

In the next chapter, we'll set about creating the new rules which will allow you to break free from your bad habits by adopting a refreshing new mindset.

6

BREAKING THE RULES

"Don't fear failure. In great attempts it is glorious even to fail"

— BRUCE LEE

Breaking free of the habits that have dictated the way you eat takes real effort. After all, you've been eating around a thousand meals a year for every year that you've been alive, so those habits are pretty well ingrained. The key to lasting change lies in undergoing a mental makeover. Unless you are able to achieve a complete mindset shift regarding food and your relationship with it, all of your actions will end up in frustration.

In this chapter, I'll provide you with a plethora of strategies, techniques and tips to allow you to develop the mindset to conquer your bad eating habits and create new rules that are guilt-free, making it far easier to maintain a healthy lifestyle.

ISSUES OF SELF ESTEEM

Research indicates that many people's bad eating habits are rooted in issues of poor self-esteem. With society's obsession with looks, that's hardly surprising. By the time the average young woman graduates from High School, she will have watched over 22,000 hours of television. That's nearly 2 and a half years of sitting in front of the TV 24 / 7. And during that time, she will have been deluged with images of sexy women with perfect bodies.

For many young women, this constant exposure to the perceived body ideal leads to a deeply seated subconscious connection between attaining a Sports illustrated Swimsuit body and love, happiness and fulfillment. And all of this has led to a distorted view of body image among many women. In a recent survey, 41% of female respondents described themselves as too fat, and 29% said that they were currently dieting. In fact, only 17% of them were overweight, according to body fat caliper testing.

The result of all of this media-fed body image control is that women have morphed their view of how they think they look onto their total self-image. A less than ideal self-body image, then, can result in some pretty toxic ideas about one's personal worth. Unless you consider yourself physically acceptable, you're likely to feel powerless, unworthy and unloved. That's pretty harsh when the view of what is acceptable is, in itself, an artificially constructed illusion. After all, the images we see in the magazines are airbrushed and photo-shopped to create an illusion of bodily perfection that simply does not exist. That's why most of us are looking at our body images through a distorted mirror. The following steps will help you to correct your view:

1. Start retraining yourself to forget about the false images that society has embedded in your brain about the body ideal. It has been designed for one thing only - to take your money. Your body is unique to you - focus on improving it bit by bit and forget everything else - and stop comparing yourself to others.
2. Judge your body by what it does for you rather than what you think it looks like. Your body is an amazing living machine that deserves your respect. Cherish it, feed it so that it can do its best and NEVER put anything into it that will cause it damage.
3. Dig to uncover the real reasons behind any ongoing body image hang-ups that you have. What is it that is really holding you back from feeling good about yourself? Could it be that you were never praised as a child? Do you expect perfection from yourself? Whatever the issue is,

make up your mind here and now to confront it rationally in the cold light of day. Acknowledge it. Accept it. Then remedy it.
4. Adopt a positive power base. You are about to engage upon an awesome weight management program that will allow you to finally achieve your physical goals. The mindset that you take into this endeavor is critical. Rather than coming from an "I'm broken and I need to be fixed" perspective, you should adopt the view that "I'm awesome and I deserve to be the best me that I can be."
5. Learn to judge yourself by what is really important. At the end of the day, your character is more important than your thigh size. Develop the qualities of love, compassion, empathy and hospitality and judge yourself against these criteria. So make a list of positive non-body traits that you appreciate about yourself. Keep this close by and refer to it every day.
6. Realize that you are not alone. Everybody has doubts about how they look - including those supermodels who you've probably been judging yourself against for so long. Without their million-dollar make-up and airbrushed photoshoots, they're just like you.
7. View yourself as a whole person - you're more than just a sagging butt or beer belly. Look at yourself naked in the mirror and focus on the bits that you do like.

8. Surround yourself with positive people who clearly love themselves and will encourage you in the same regard. These people should love you for who you are, not what you have or how you look.
9. Be stronger than your negative thoughts. Shut them down, boot them out and clear the space for positivity. Any time you see a negative thought taking root, squash it and put a positive affirmation in its place.
10. Treat your body. Take a soothing bubble bath. Have a relaxing nap. Just find some time to chill out. Give back to the body that, up until now, you've probably been berating and taking for granted.

UNDERSTANDING HUNGER

In order to break the bad eating habits that have accumulated over your life, you need to really understand what hunger is, what contributes to true hunger and how to differentiate between physical and emotional hunger.

When your stomach is empty of food, you experience hunger pangs in the form of contractions of the stomach wall. However, these stomach contractions are not only caused by lack of food. They may also occur as the result of your body's rhythms. The human body thrives on regularity and over the years, each of us has trained our body to eat at certain times. When we miss one of those feeding times, the body may react to physical cues like stomach contractions even though we are not busy.

The body's intake of food is regulated by two key hormones:

- Leptin
- Ghrelin

Leptin: The Hunger Controller

Leptin is one of the body's master hormones. Among its many other roles, leptin has the job of controlling how hungry you feel. This hormone is released by your fat cells and keeps a constant tally on your stored fat content and the amount of food you need to consume to provide the energy you need to function.

The higher the levels of leptin circulating through your system, the lower the levels of a hunger signaling hormone called NPY. A rodent study conducted by the Rockefeller Institute found that obese mice who were injected with leptin had a significantly reduced food intake and a boosted fat burn.

Research like this has led scientists to proclaim leptin as the 'gate-keeper of fat metabolism and the regulator of hunger'. As well as negating the hunger-boosting effects of NPY, it has also been shown to counter the hunger-stimulating effects of another hormone called anandamide. In addition, leptin is believed to stimulate the body's production of a hormone called a-MSH, which acts as an appetite suppressant.

When your body produces a normal level of leptin, the brain will receive appropriate messages to stop eating when you are full and you will be able to control your appetite. Because leptin is produced in our fat cells, the more stored body fat we have, the more leptin we will produce. You'd think that this will help overweight people to eat less. However, there's a problem.

When your body is overwhelmed by leptin production due to too many stored fat cells, you can develop what is known as leptin resistance. This is when the brain fails to respond to the signals it is receiving to stop eating. It has been overwhelmed by the hormone and metaphorically throws up its hands in despair. As a result, the body reverts to its starvation response of eating more and exercising less to preserve energy.

The following factors contribute to leptin resistance:

- eating too many simple carbohydrates
- high-stress levels
- high fructose
- overconsumption of grain
- lack of sleep

To avoid leptin resistance, be sure to follow these guidelines:

- Establish a sleep routine
- Get up at the same time each day
- Limit daytime napping:
- Get a handle on stress
- Cut down the coffee and alcohol
- Keep all technology out of your bedroom, including your smartphone
- Reduce your intake of sugar and processed carbohydrates
- Eat a protein with every meal
- Eat more healthy fats such as coconut oil, avocado and fish oil
- Eat your dinner 2-3 hours before bed time
- Perform high-intensity interval training (HIIT) workout 2-3 times per week

Ghrelin: The Hunger Initiator

Ghrelin is the yin to leptin's yang; it signals hunger while leptin signals fullness. Ghrelin is produced in an upper part of the stomach called the fundus. Its production increases when we are genuinely hungry. But hunger is not the only thing that leads to increased ghrelin secretion. So does lack of sleep. Research has even shown that simply looking at images of temping foods leads to enhanced ghrelin production.

Here are 3 ways to reduce ghrelin levels:

- Increase your intake of high fiber foods
- Eat lean protein at every meal

- Get 7-8 hours of sleep each night

THE TEN TYPES OF HUNGER

According to dietitians, there are 10 different types of hunger, each of which has a specific way to keep it in check. Let's consider each one briefly:

Eye Hunger

There's a reason why the most popular item pictured on Instagram is food; we eat with our eyes! When we see a beautifully presented food item, we feel an overwhelming urge to eat it immediately. I bet even looking at the front cover of this book made you want to go out and buy a candy bar!

> The Solution: Stop looking - immediately divert your focus to a non-food item that brings you pleasure.

Ear Hunger

Hearing food, or simply hearing about it, can set our mouth to watering and make us feel that we simply must have that food now. It could be something as innocent as a person opening a packet of potato chips on the train or a delivery guy announcing Pizza's arrival next door.

> The Solution: Again, the solution is to discipline your mind to divert your attention to something

else that will consume you and make you forget that false hunger cue.

Nose Hunger

Food sellers have been using the enticing smell of food for hundreds of years. Whether it's freshly baked banana bread, an oven-baked lasagna or freshly brewed coffee, that irresistible odor seems to entrance us, destroying our willpower and causing us to succumb to those temptations.

> The Solution: Make the effort to individually smell all of the foods on your plate. Take in the odor of each food as you consume it. When you do this, you will be teaching yourself to slow down, eat more mindfully and, as a result, you will eat less food overall.

Stomach Hunger

When your stomach is empty, it will 'growl' to let you know that it needs food. However, as previously mentioned, this stomach growling can also be due to the body's adherence to an established eating schedule rather than legitimate hunger.

> The Solution: Use the Hunger Gauge that was introduced earlier to assess your actual as opposed to your perceived hunger level. Slow down in your

eating and leave the table when you are not quite full.

Mouth Hunger

Mouth hunger is controlled by the taste buds. They create an intense desire for certain foods. These cravings are not a sign of actual hunger. However, they can be almost impossible to resist.

> The Solution: Satisfy the craving with a small portion. When you do that, the craving will disappear. That is when you need to discipline yourself to stop.

Heart Hunger

Heart hunger can also be termed emotional hunger, where we eat for psychological rather than physical reasons.

> The Solution: Practice the mindful eating strategies we have already considered. Reduce portion sizes and, once again, use the Hunger Gauge to assess your real state of hunger.

Cellular Hunger

Leptin and Ghrelin, introduced in the previous section, are the cellular controllers of appetite. The heavier a person is, however, the out of balance these hormones become in favor of Ghrelin, the hunger initiator.

The Solution: Control your food regulating hormones by getting 7-8 hours sleep each night, eating lean protein at every meal and increasing fiber intake.

Stress Hunger

When we are stressed, we eat for comfort. Our minds are consumed without problems, so we don't have the energy to regulate what we are putting into our mouths. Rather, we eat for comfort.

The Solution: Pause and force yourself to think of the consequences of your stress-induced food choices. Will they make you feel guilty later? Will you end up with a bloated stomach, gas and bloating? Is that what you really need?

Midnight Hunger

Many people wake during the night with a strong urge to go to the fridge and break open a tub of ice cream or pound back an extra-large piece of chocolate cake. This may be stress-related or a result of hormonal imbalance in favor of Ghrelin.

The Solution: Follow the sleep tips already given to increase the chances of not waking in the middle of the night. In case you do, have a small healthy snack on the bedside table, such as a handful of almonds or a banana.

Thirst Hunger

This last type of hunger should really be called mistaken hunger. We think we are hungry when we are, in fact, thirsty. The body triggers its sensation for food and water based on diminished energy levels. These two sensations reach the brain together – and most people interpret them to be a sensation just to eat. The body does not send a separate signal for thirst and another one for food. As a result, we often reach for food when we should be reaching for water.

> The Solution: Drink a glass of water before you eat. When you do that, you will satisfy the body's need for hydration and you will prevent yourself from overeating.

3 STRATEGIES FOR ADOPTING HEALTHY EATING HABITS

From a psychological point of view, it is also more advantageous to add than to subtract. When it comes to your eating habits, thinking in terms of adding positive habits rather than getting rid of negative ones will put you at an advantage. Of course, in the process of adopting the good, you will be dropping the bad.

Here are three strategies that have been identified by psychologists when adopting healthy eating habits . . .

Manage Your Expectations

Many people set unrealistic expectations around their new eating goals. For one thing, they may expect to lose weight a lot faster than is realistic. The only thing that you should want to lose is stored body fat. A consistent weight loss of 1-2 pounds per week is realistic.

Aside from the drop in scale weight, people often have unrealistic emotional expectations. They may think that losing weight will bring them happiness. Yet, happiness is a multi-faceted diamond. Losing weight may contribute to that state but it will not assure it. However, if that is your expectation, there is a high chance that, when you don't find it, you will give up on your new eating habits and revert back to your old ways.

As a result, it is important to make your expectations about your new eating habits realistic.

Set Realistic Goals

Pressuring yourself with too many goals around your eating habits is a sure way to failure. The key to success is to slowly yet steadily implement one change at a time. Don't introduce a new habit until you have got on top of the previous one.

Focus on Adding, Not Removing, Foods

When you remove anything, you can't help but have a slight feeling of deprivation. Avoid this by concentrating on adding healthy foods to your day rather than excluding unhealthy foods. If you introduce the habit of having a mid-morning snack of sliced apple and walnuts, for example, you will, without focusing on it, have removed the habit of chowing down on cookies as your snack of choice.

Get Back on the Horse

Never forget that you are a human being, not a robot. Your progress toward healthy eating will not be linear. There will be setbacks and there will be times when you feel like a failure. Realizing and accepting that at the outset is critical to success.

When you slip up and revert to eating the way you know you shouldn't, you need to isolate that episode and move on from it. Don't beat yourself up over your slip-up. Simply accept it, get back on the horse and keep moving forward.

HOW HABITS WORK

Let's conclude this chapter with a consideration of how habits are formed. This will allow you to strategically use each of the habit formation stages as the basis for adding new habits and dismantling old ones. I'll then provide you with a dozen habits that you should begin to adopt at any age, but especially if you are over the age of 40.

There are three steps to the creation of habits:

1. The Trigger
2. The Behavior
3. The Reward

The Trigger

Everything starts with the habit trigger. You need to take the time to initiate the right triggers. There are four main types of triggers that cure our habits:

Location

Our environment has a powerful effect on our actions. By manipulating your environment in favor of a desirable outcome, you will be far more likely to follow through with the habit you are trying to introduce. For example, you will be more likely to introduce the habit of eating more fruit as a snack by purchasing beautiful fresh fruit every few days and displaying it on your kitchen counter than if you allow the bananas to go black and mushy and hardly ever top up your apple and citrus supply.

Time

Connect your new habit to a certain time of the day. You probably already have a set time to get up in the morning. Let's stay it is 6:30am. If you are trying to introduce the habit of drinking more water, tie the habit to the clock so that at 6:35am you drink a full glass of water. You might not feel like drinking water at that time but you will do it anyway because you know that is what your body needs and you are regulated by the clock.

Prior Actions

Connecting a habit to a prior action is known as habit stacking. It involves introducing a new habit by piggybacking off another habit or routine that you have already ingrained in your life. For example, you may have the routine of walking to the bus each morning. If you are trying to develop the habit of eating more fruit, pair it with grabbing an apple on your way out the door.

The Actions of Others

Other people have a huge influence on our actions and our habits. As far as it depends upon you, surround yourself with people who are also trying to eat in a more healthy manner. Explain the reasons for your desire to break your bad eating habits to your loved ones and ask for their support. Even if they don't fully embrace your new ways of eating, knowing that they are behind and will not do things to jeopardize your goals makes a big difference.

The Behavior

The behavior or 'action' is simply the response to these triggers. As previously stated, if you use the correct triggers, you are likely to follow up with the intended behavior. For example, if you display fresh fruit in the kitchen, you are far more likely to eat it than if it is hidden away in the fridge. You are also using healthier foods like fresh fruit and nuts as a replacement to snacking on processed, high sugar treats. If you don't buy these unhealthy foods at the store, you are limiting your chances of eating them on a regular basis.

The Reward

The habit reward stage is built on the established principle of operant conditioning, which states that, if we receive a positive feeling after doing something, we will continue doing it. When it comes to adopting your nutritional habits, you will feel immediate psychological rewards in terms of feeling better about yourself and your ability to master nutritional temptation. Allow yourself to go there mentally, congratulating yourself for what you are achieving. You will also experience improved physical health almost immediately. You will feel less bloated, sluggish and weighted down. Problems you may have had with gas and acid reflux will begin to lessen and you will start to lose those extra pounds. Recognize and acknowledge these rewards for your actions.

Your brain will soon understand that if it sees the cue and does the action, it will get the reward. When you think about it, switching from a bad habit to a good habit doesn't have to require changing all three of these steps. If you stick with the same trigger and reward but simply switch out the action in the middle, you should, theoretically, be able to transform a bad habit into a good habit.

Let's consider an example to see how this might work in practice:

> *You're at work and it comes to your lunch break. Everyone else automatically heads outside for a cigarette break. But you are trying to break the smoking habit, you head out for a 10 minute walk in the fresh air.*

We see that the cue remains the same- the lunch bell. The activity changes. But the reward, getting out of the work environment and relaxing the mind remains the same. You also get the extra benefit of fresh air, which you can't exactly claim on a cigarette break!

CHANGING A BAD HABIT TO A GOOD HABIT

Let's stick with the bad habit of smoking to analyze the change process in a little more detail.

There are all sorts of cues for a person to light up a cigarette. These might include going outside, being stressed or just being bored. The first step to conquering your bad habit is to write down all of the cues that lead you to reach for a cigarette.

Next, you need to find a replacement habit that is somewhat similar but better for you. An example would be to pop a piece of gum into your mouth. This makes sense when it comes to defeating the smoking habit because research tells us that the smoking habit has a lot to do with the fixation on the mouth. You are breathing in and out and holding the cigarette between your lips. So, replacing it with an activity that is also mouth-centric, like chewing gum, makes sense.

The replacement activity needs to also provide a reward. This might require a bit of thinking. You need to be careful because people often replace one bad habit with another. A common one is to go from smoking to eating.

This results in excess calorie consumption and weight gain.

One strategy that you could utilize is to put aside the money that you would have previously spent on cigarettes to provide a tangible reward. If you used to smoke a pack of cigarettes a day, at an average cost of $6.50 per pack, that's a little under $50 a week that you'll be able to put aside. Maybe you can take your partner out for a restaurant meal once a fortnight or go out for a movie. Even though the reward will not be immediate when you are replacing the habit, it will still be powerful to provide the positive reinforcement that you need to succeed.

A DOZEN NUTRITIONAL CHANGES TO EMBRACE BEFORE YOU TURN 40

When you move into your fourth decade, your body's nutritional needs change. That's because you are now dealing with the effects of age-related hormonal and physical changes that are occurring inside your body. The following 12 healthy changes to adopt in your 40s come directly from the top doctors, nutritionists and mental health professionals on the planet. Remember to add them one at a time and not to move on to the next one until the current habit is ingrained.

Change #1: Avoid blood sugar spikes by snacking on lean protein, nuts and fruit as an energy pick-me-up rather than processed high glycemic carb foods.

Change #2: Cut your caffeine consumption back to between 50-80 mg per day; that's the equivalent of one medium-sized cup of coffee. Replace your other previous coffee breaks with water.

Change #3: Start supplementing with fish oil and a daily multivitamin that contains at least 2.4 mcg of Vitamin B12.

Change #4: Cut out empty calories; your body can no longer get away with several portions of junk each week! After 40 you need to make smarter choices about how you fuel your body. Go for the most nutrient-dense foods that provide maximum value for the minimum caloric cost.

Change #5: Plan to eat 20-30 grams of protein per meal. That will fill you up and help offset age-related muscle wasting.

Change #6: Consciously think about getting more antioxidants in the form of vegetables, fruits, nuts and beans.

Change #7: Increase your intake of omega-3 fatty acids by including eggs, fatty fish, nuts and avocados in your diet.

Change #8: Set a priority on including high fiber foods in your diet. This will help with digestion and elimination as well as keeping you regular. Fiber also fills the stomach so that you are less likely to graze between meals.

Change #9: Look after your bone health by including 3 servings of dairy per day. This will provide you with about 1000 mg of calcium. If you are vegan or don't do well with dairy, get your calcium from sweet potatoes, baby carrots, green beans, broccoli and oranges.

Change #10: Reduce your plate size. Go down from 12 inches to 9 inch diameter plates and your daily caloric consumption will reduce by a quarter!

Change #11: Start a Food Journal. This is a great way to keep yourself accountable and to begin thinking mindfully about what you are eating and why. If you get into the habit of recording everything you've eaten in the early evening, you will also be far less likely to eat rubbish food before going to bed.

Change #12: Strength Training. Beginning a regular, balanced strength training program before the age of 40 will allow you to face the future head-on. Strength training has been shown to be effective at combating every single one of the biomarkers of aging. Research also shows that people who are regularly exercising are far more likely to be successful at making long-term positive changes to the way they eat.

SUMMARY

In this chapter, we have established the mental foundation to break bad eating habits and adopt new, healthier nutritional habits. We identified issues of self-esteem as being at the root of many people's poor eating habits and then provided 10 strategies to improve self-esteem and break away from society's body obsession.

We then took a deep dive into what true hunger is and how to differentiate between physical and emotional hunger. We identified the two key hormones that regulate hunger...

- Leptin
- Ghrelin

In order to balance these key hormones, you need to:

- Get 7-8 hours of sleep each night
- Eat protein with every meal
- Do High-Intensity Interval Training (HIIT) Workouts
- Eat more high-fiber foods

We then identified the 10 types of hunger as identified by dietitians along with strategies to control each of them. Next, we focused on strategies for adopting healthy eating habits, including managing expectations, setting realistic goals and focusing on adding rather than removing foods and getting back on track when you slip up.

The three parts of the Habit Loop were identified...

- The Trigger
- The Behaviour
- The Reward

… and I showed you how they can be used to change a bad habit into a good habit.

We concluded this chapter with a dozen nutritional changes that everyone by the age of 40 should embrace.

In the next chapter, we focus on the importance of food as energy, as well the vital role that hydration and recovery play in combating many of the factors that contribute to bad eating habits.

STEP THREE. PRACTICAL SOLUTIONS

7

FUEL, HYDRATION & RECOVERY

> *"Your body is your most priceless possession. Take care of it"*
>
> — JACK LALANE

Without energy, you will not survive. The one and only source of that life-giving fuel is food. That food comes into your body in the form of three macro, or large, nutrients:

- Carbohydrates
- Proteins
- Fats

As those fuel sources are digested in the body, they are broken down into glucose, amino acids and fatty acids. These compounds enter the bloodstream and are then utilized in the process of respiration, which creates adenosine triphosphate (ATP), the main fuel that our bodies use.

There are three ways that the body creates ATP. These three energy systems are:

- The ATP-PCR system
- The glycolytic system
- The oxidative system

The first two of these energy systems do not require oxygen, while the third one does. As a result, it is also known as the aerobic (literally 'living in air') system.

The ATP-PCR system allows for exercise between 5-15 seconds. The ATP stored in the muscle will power up to the first five seconds. The salt phosphate (PCR) attaches to ATP to provide another 10 seconds or so of energy.

Once the ATP-PCR system is used up, the body switches to the glycolytic system. Now the body relies upon glycogen, which is the broken-down form of carbohydrate, to make ATP. This is achieved through the process of glycolysis. During glycolysis, lactate is produced, along with hydrogen ions. These are responsible for the muscle burn and fatigue you feel when sprinting or lifting heavy weights.

The glycolytic system will sustain you for up to two minutes of exercise. After that, the body switches to the oxidative system. With this system, ATP is produced using two mechanisms:

- The Krebs cycle
- The electron transport chain

The oxidative system produces ATP more slowly than the other two systems, but it will provide energy for a greater duration. This explains why you can run slowly for a long period of time, but sprint for only a short period of time, before you are exhausted.

SPOTLIGHT ON THE MACRONUTRIENTS

The amount of energy stored in food is measured in calories. In terms of the macronutrients:

- Carbohydrates contain 4 calories per gram
- Proteins contain 4 calories per gram
- Fats contain 9 calories per gram

As a guide, the average adult male needs 2500 calories daily and, and the average woman needs 2000 calories daily to maintain a healthy weight. This amount will vary depending on how much you exercise (you will require fewer calories if you are sedentary than if you are very active).

Along with providing energy, all of these macronutrients have specific roles in your body that allow you to function properly.

Carbohydrates

Carbohydrates (or carbs) are the only one of the three macronutrients that are not essential for life. Though the glucose which it provides is essential, this can also be obtained from fats and proteins. Getting glucose from carbs, though, is faster and more efficient.

Carbohydrates can be classified as either simple or complex. Simple carbs are quickly absorbed into the body. They cause an immediate surge in blood glucose levels. This effect is pronounced when you eat carbs by themselves, which is one reason you should avoid doing this. The rate at which carbohydrates are absorbed and digested has a direct bearing on energy levels, body composition and overall health. Carbs that are 'time-released' from low glycemic index foods will keep you fuller for longer, balance out your blood sugar and provide a slow release of energy.

Carbohydrates with a low glycemic-index are found in vegetables, fruits, legumes, and whole grains and should predominate in the diet over simple carbs such as fruit, dairy products, and processed and refined sugars like candy, table sugar, syrups, and soft drinks.

Neither simple nor complex carbs are good or bad. However, your dietary focus should be on complex carbs, with simple carbs being reserved as sometimes or treat foods.

Complex carbs don't provide the immediate energy that you get with simple carbs. But nor do they cause havoc with your blood sugar levels. They are more substantial and filling than simple carbs and usually contain fiber, which is a form of carbohydrate that is indigestible to humans and is extremely important for our gut health.

Complex carbs can be further divided into starches and fibrous vegetables.

Plants store energy in the form of starch. The following are the most common starchy foods that you should include in your diet:

- Yams
- Whole Grains
- Bread
- Pulses
- Beans
- Corn
- Pumpkin
- Sweet Potatoes

Because the human body can digest all of the calorie energy in starchy carbs, they are said to be more calorie-dense than fibrous carbs.

It is vital, however, that a healthy nutrition plan includes a healthy supply of fibrous vegetables. Here are some common types of fibrous carbs that should also feature on your plate regularly:

- Broccoli
- Asparagus
- Cauliflower
- Spinach
- Lettuce
- Brussels sprouts
- Tomatoes
- Cucumber
- Peppers
- Onions
- Bok choy
- Kale
- Mushrooms
- Courgettes

Fats

Fats are organic molecules that are made of carbon and hydrogen. They join together in long chains called hydrocarbons. The way that these hydrocarbons form and their length determines the type of fat that is created.

The simplest unit of fat is the fatty acid. Depending on the number of hydrogens affixed to each carbon along the hydrocarbon chain, two different types of fatty acids are formed:

- Saturated

- Unsaturated

The difference between saturated and unsaturated fatty acids comes down to their bond structure. Saturated fatty acids do not contain any double bonds and they have a full complement of hydrogen molecules associated with each carbon molecule.

Unsaturated fatty acids do contain double bonds and have fewer hydrogen molecules. They are able to be broken down into monounsaturated fatty acids, in which only one carbon is unsaturated, and polyunsaturated fatty acids, in which more than one carbon is unsaturated.

Fatty acids can be joined together to form what is known as triglycerides. This occurs when three fatty acids join together with a glycerol molecule. Triglycerides are the main component of fat in the diet. They are also the major form of storage fat on the body.

Saturated fats are found mainly in animal-based foods, whereas unsaturated fats are predominant in plant-based foods.

Because many people eat a lot of animal-based foods and few plant-based foods, they have an imbalance in favor of saturated fats. This is often combined with a high carbohydrate intake, which appears to accentuate the ill effects of a high saturated fat intake. It is recommended that our unsaturated to saturated fat intake ratio should be around 65:35.

Common sources of saturated fats include:

- Meat
- Poultry
- Butter
- Cheese
- Palm Oils

When we consume fats, the process of digestion involves the breaking down of triglycerides into fatty acids and glycerol. The fatty acids are an important source of energy for the body. In fact, a gram of fat has more than twice the energy potential of a gram of carbohydrate. Fats are also used for the manufacture and balance of hormones, the formation of cell membranes, and fat-soluble vitamins A, D, E and K.

Proteins

Every part of your body, from your big toe to the hairs on your head, is constructed from protein. Proteins are made up of chains of amino acids. The quality of a protein depends on its completeness according to its amino acid profile. There are 20 amino acids that are needed by the human body for growth. These 20 amino acids form into an untold number of configurations to make all manner of molecules. Eleven of the twenty can be manufactured within the human body.

That leaves nine amino acids that have to come from the foods we eat. These are the essential amino acids:

- Histidine
- Isoleucine
- Leucine
- Valine
- Lysine
- Methionine
- Phenylalanine
- Threonine
- Tryptophan

Animal protein sources, such as meat, fish, poultry, eggs, milk and cheese, are considered to be complete proteins. There are some plant protein sources that are also complete in their amino acid profile. These include:

- Quinoa
- Buckwheat
- Hempseed
- Amaranth

Most plant sources of protein, however, are considered to be incomplete because they do not contain all of the essential amino acids. In order to get all of the essential amino acids, people who follow a plant-based nutrition plan should use complementary protein choices. Combining wheat or rice, which are limited in lysine, with legumes, which are limited in tryptophan, can provide a full essential amino acid intake.

Water

Your body thrives on water. We use water in every cell, organ and tissue in order to maintain our body functions. In fact, according to the US Geological Survey, 60% of your body is water. To put that another way, if you're a 150-pound man, 90 of those pounds (40 liters) are water!

Water has many roles in the body, including:

- Regulating body temperature
- Lubricating joints
- Moistening tissues for mouth, eyes and nose
- Protecting body organs and tissues
- Preventing constipation
- Helping dissolve minerals and other nutrients to make them accessible to the body
- Reducing the burden on the kidneys and liver by flushing out waste products
- Carrying nutrients and oxygen to the cells

Without the right amount of water, your body simply will not function properly. However, we lose water just by going about our daily lives. If our 150 lb man does nothing all day except sit and breathe, he will still lose around 1.5 L of water over the course of the day through sweating, urination, and respiration. The more activity he does, the more water he will lose. If he does not replace this water, he will become dehydrated.

Dehydration reduces the amount of blood in the body, forcing the heart to pump harder in order to deliver oxygen-bearing cells into our muscles. For our 150 lb man, losing 3-5 L (just 1/8 of his body's water) of water will result in headaches and lethargy. After losing 6-7 L of water, mental impairments become apparent. If he loses much more than 10 L, he will go into shock and die. It is therefore vitally important that water lost is replenished.

So, how do you meet your daily hydration needs?

You have probably heard the often-cited recommendation to consume 8 glasses of water per day. That is a good guideline to aim for. The best way to meet that goal is to carry a water bottle with you and regularly sip from it, with the goal of getting through two and a half 750 ml (25 oz) bottles over the course of the day.

THE IMPORTANCE OF SLEEP

You enter your bedroom, change into your pajamas and slip between the sheets. You snuggle into the fetal position, each muscle in your body loosening and relaxing and your mind emptying. Your head sinks into the comfort of your pillow as you relish this time of recuperation – your daily reward for a hard day's work. You close your eyes and drift into a peaceful, regenerative sleep.

In those moments before you fall asleep, melatonin is produced in your brain. Its job is to slow down your metabolism. As melatonin begins coursing through your body, your body temperature drops slightly, blood flow to the brain is reduced and your muscles slowly start to loosen and become flaccid.

You now gently move into the first stage of what is known as non-REM or non-Dream sleep. This is shallow sleep during which your brain waves perform in rapid, irregular patterns. Your muscles become totally relaxed and your metabolism slows further as more melatonin is released. You will go through this first stage several times during the course of the evening. Each one will last between 30 seconds and seven minutes.

You now cruise straight into stage two, which has been called true sleep. About 20% of your night will be spent in this stage. It is characterized by enlarged brain waves as your mind produces fragmented ideas and visuals. Yet you are in a deep sleep and have no awareness of your surroundings.

Stages three and four are known as the delta zone. You are moving from deeper into deepest sleep. During this phase, the majority of the blood coursing around your body is being directed to your muscles. Your brain produces enlarged, slow waves. You are now in the power stage of sleep. Someone trying to wake you would have the most difficulty during stage four sleep. That's because it's during this phase that your body is replenishing, recovering and repairing itself. Ideally, you will spend about 50% of the night in stage four sleep.

About two hours into your slumber, your eyes will start to quiver rapidly backward and forwards. You are entering what scientists have dubbed Rapid Eye Movement (REM) sleep. Researchers have discovered that during a good night's sleep, you will move in and out of the REM stage several times. It is during REM sleep that you dream, as more blood is redirected to your brain. In fact, during REM your brain is acting almost as if you were awake.

Throughout the night, you are constantly moving through the 5 stages of sleep – the four non-REM stages and REM – such that every 90 minutes you are in REM sleep. Each time you enter REM, however, the phase lasts longer.

After seven to eight hours of uninterrupted sleep, you will go through six or seven complete sleep cycles. You will wake up refreshed, invigorated and ready to seize the coming day.

The Consequences of Broken Sleep

It should be clear from the above that several portions of broken sleep do not add up to the same amount of uninterrupted sleep. If you are waking up several times during the night, you may not be giving yourself enough time to reach stage four non-REM or REM sleep. Then, when – and if – you drift back to sleep again, you start back at Phase One again. That's why people who suffer from broken sleep can suffer from fatigue, apathy and depression the next day.

When you are regularly denied the cyclical 5 phases of sleep, you develop what is called **sleep debt**. Sleep debt prevents you from getting the amount of REM sleep that you need. REM sleep is vital for mental health. Bodily repair takes place during Stage 4 of non-REM sleep. Without these vital repair stages, you will suffer from:

- Reduced attention span
- Memory and vocabulary loss
- Diminished analytical thinking ability
- Diminished creativity
- A diminished sense of humor and social skills
- Reduced communication and decision skills
- Diminished resistance to viruses
- Reduced work productivity
- Enhanced risk-taking
- Increased likelihood of heart attack
- Increased susceptibility to diabetes
- Increased susceptibility to cold and flu
- Increased irritability
- Fat gain
- General lethargy
- Fatigue
- Lack of interest in what is going on around you

That is quite an ominous list. However, many people who are accustomed to getting by on a minimum amount of sleep are not even aware of many of these effects. Even though constant sleep shortage may diminish their mental faculties – specifically their alertness and reaction time – they operate under the mistaken impression that they haven't been affected at all. One result of this deceptive thinking can be seen in the carnage that occurs every day on our motorways.

Establishing Good Bedtime Habits

Clear Out Bedroom Junk

Your bedroom should be for two things only - sleep and sex. If you have TV in the bedroom, or you take your phone to bed with you, you will be tempted to use them, causing havoc to your sleep plans.

Establish a Wind-Down Routine

If you go to bed with your head buzzing and your stomach still trying to digest your last meal, you are going to struggle to get to sleep. A wind-down routine that begins a few hours ahead of hitting the sack can make all the difference.

Plan to finish your last meal three hours before going to bed. Then, about an hour and a half before going to bed, find something soothing to do in dim light. You could read a book, listen to music, work on a jigsaw puzzle, or anything else that you find calming and relaxing.

Follow your relaxing hour up with a warm bath. Stay in the water for at least ten minutes and get out at least an hour before bedtime. This will allow your core body temperature to cool down.

With half an hour to go before bedtime, fill out a 'To-Do' journal, in which you write down everything you need to do the next day. This will mean that you will spend less time agonizing about what you need to be doing the next day in the middle of the night.

Eating Your Way to a Good Night's Sleep

Changing what and when you eat can help you to get a better night's sleep. Here are the key facts you need to know:

- Do not eat within, ideally, three hours of bedtime.
- Cut back on sugar, sugary treats, drinks and desserts, particularly shop-bought ones.
- Get more fiber into your diet by switching to brown rice and by eating more quinoa, bulgar, whole rye, wholegrain barley, wild rice, buckwheat, lentils and beans.
- Full-fat yogurt is a good source of probiotics. Add blackberries, strawberries or blueberries for flavor and sprinkle in some walnuts.
- Eat such oily fish as salmon, tuna, and mackerel, which are rich in omega-3 fatty acids, two to three times per week.

SUMMARY

In this chapter, we have focused on the biological reason we eat, which is to provide the energy needed to power us through our lives. We've discovered that adenosine triphosphate (ATP) is the primary fuel that our bodies use. There are 3 ways that the body manufactures ATP:

- The ATP-PCR system
- The glycolytic system

- The oxidative system

We then shone a spotlight on the 3 key macronutrients. Carbohydrates, which provide glucose, are the most efficient energy source. Carbs also provide fiber, which promotes satiety and boosts gut health.

Fats can be either saturated or unsaturated. Fats, in the form of triglycerides, are the major form of fat storage in the body. Protein, in the form of amino acids, makes up the building material of the body. Humans cannot manufacture 9 of the 20 amino acids that are most crucial to the body. Foods that contain all 9 of the essential amino acids are known as complete proteins.

Finally, we touched on hydration and rest. Water is essential to the efficient functioning of the body – you should aim to drink 8 glasses of water each day. Sleep is also crucial to overall health, being especially important for renewing energy levels and relieving stress.

8

SO, WHAT SHOULD MY MEALS LOOK LIKE?

"Your diet is like a bank account. Good food choices are good investments"

— BETHENNY FRANKEL

We now come to the part of this book where the rubber meets the road. Having gone in-depth on the bad eating habits that develop over our lives, and then provided the strategies to break free of those habits, we are able to zero in on the nutritional habits that will revolutionize the way you eat and transform your energy levels, your health and the way your body looks and feels.

Over the past half-century, various governmental agencies around the world have released a number of nutritional templates, each of which was lauded as the best way for everyone to eat. The USDA Food Pyramid was introduced in 1992 and eagerly adopted across the nation. Unfortunately, its advice was seriously flawed as the result of agricultural business lobbying.

This food pyramid was based on the premise that all carbohydrates are good for our health. That is why carb-based foods such as bread and pasta formed the wide base of the pyramid. At the other end of the pyramid, representing its narrow tip, were fats, which were to be consumed sparingly. However, it wasn't long before researchers began to identify issues with this advice. A variety of updates have been made in the official US Dietary Guidelines since then, and current guidance suggests following Harvard's Healthy Eating Plate. This is a colorful plate-shaped graphic created by Harvard Health Publishing, a division of Harvard Medical School, and is based on the most up-to-date nutritional research. It has the added benefit that it is not influenced by food industry or agriculture policy and is the way that I would recommend trying to eat on a daily basis.

The Healthy Eating Plate is divided into four unequal-sized sections:

- The largest section is **green** for vegetables
- Two-quarters of the plate are **orange** for protein and **brown** for whole grains
- The smallest section is **red** for fruits

In addition to the plate, there is a glass representing water, a bottle representing healthy plant oils, and a running figure representing exercise. The guidance suggests that you skip sugary drinks entirely, limit milk and dairy products to a maximum of two servings daily, and fruit juice to one small glass per day.

Let's take a closer look at the foods that make up each of these sections.

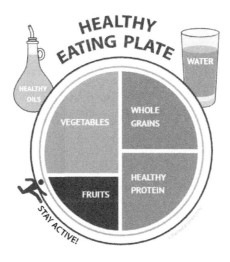

PLANT-BASED FOODS: VEGETABLES, WHOLE GRAINS & FRUITS

As the Healthy Eating Plate suggests, plants should form the basis of your diet. Both fruit and vegetables contain the vitamins, minerals, and other micronutrients that your body needs in order to run in tip-top condition! Plus, the trillions of microbes living in our gut (known as our gut microbiome, which is essential in helping to control digestion and boosting your immune system) require different types of plant foods to thrive. Increasing the diversity of the plant-based foods we eat helps to strengthen our gut microbiome, which in turn results in better health!

Furthermore, plant-based foods are naturally high in fiber. Though not officially classified as essential, fiber is an extremely important nutrient. There are two forms of fiber; soluble and insoluble.

Soluble fiber is found in such foods as oats and oat bran, dried beans and peas, nuts, barley, flax, fruits like oranges and apples, and carrots. Insoluble fiber is found in vegetables such as green beans and dark green leafy vegetables, fruit skins and root vegetable skins, whole-wheat products, seeds, and nuts. Both types of fiber, while indigestible, play important dietary roles:

- Fiber slows down the breakdown of carbohydrates into glucose. This helps to balance

out blood sugar levels and prevent sharp spikes in insulin release.
- Fiber helps us feel fuller for longer by slowing down the release of hunger-promoting hormones.
- Soluble fiber helps to reduce unhealthy cholesterol levels.
- Insoluble fiber adds bulk to stools and decreases colonic transit time, which helps to boost our overall gut health.

Plus, an increase of just 8 g of fiber per day has been linked with:

- 19% reduction in risk of heart disease.
- 15% reduction in risk of type 2 diabetes.
- 8% lower risk of colon cancer.

Though the minimum recommended intake for fiber is 25 grams per day, the optimal amount seems to be closer to 35 grams per day for women and 48 grams per day for men.

However, just 10% of us are getting the recommended amount of fiber daily!

So, how do we ensure we get adequate plant diversity on our plate?

You may have heard of the World Health Organisation's recommendation of '5 A Day', as eating 400 g of fruit and vegetables (or five portions of fruit and veg) has been shown to lower the risk of serious health problems such as heart disease, stroke, and even some forms of cancer. In 2021 research conducted by at Harvard T. H. Chan School of Public Health found that eating two servings of fruit and three servings of vegetables is associated with lower mortality rates.

Furthermore, researchers at King's College London have also suggested that all fruits, veggies, wholegrains, legumes (beans and pulses), nuts and seeds, and herbs and spices count to this total!

Here are some tips to help you increase your plant-based foods intake:

- Always choose whole grains over refined grains, which have been stripped of valuable nutrients (including fiber) during processing. This could be as simple as switching from white to wholegrain bread, keeping the skin on your vegetables when cooking, or sprinkling seeds onto your salads.
- Place fruit where you can see it, e.g. in a bowl on the kitchen counter, or chopped up (fruit salad style) in a bowl in the fridge.
- Go exploring down the produce aisle and regularly try new vegetables.
- Aim to eat the rainbow!

Add Color to Your Plate with the Food Rainbow

Filling your plate with a variety of colors does more than look good. Each of those colors represents a different nutrient profile that nourishes and enriches your body. Make it your aim to include two to three colors on your plate at each meal.

Here are the key foods to consume in each color range and the key nutrients they provide:

Red

- Tomatoes
- Pink Guava
- Grapefruit
- Red Bell Peppers

Key Nutrients: Lycopene, Folate, Potassium, Vitamin C, Vitamin B6

Orange and Yellow

- Carrots
- Sweet Potatoes
- Yellow Bell Peppers
- Bananas
- Pineapple
- Tangerines
- Pumpkin
- Winter Squash
- Corn

Key Nutrients: Carotenoids, Fiber, Folate, Potassium, Vitamin A, Vitamin C

Green

- Spinach
- Kale
- Broccoli
- Asparagus
- Avocados
- Green Cabbage
- Brussels Sprouts
- Green Herbs
- Green Bell Peppers

Key Nutrients: Chlorophyll, Carotenoids, Indoles, Fiber, Folate, Iron, Potassium, Vitamin A, Vitamin K1, Vitamin C, Vitamin B6

Blue & Purple

- Blueberries
- Blackberries
- Concord Grapes
- Red/Purple Cabbage
- Eggplant
- Plums
- Elderberries

Key Nutrients: Anthocyanins, Fiber, Manganese, Potassium, Vitamin B6, Vitamin C, Vitamin K1

Dark Red

- Beets
- Prickly Pears

Key Nutrients: Betalains, Fiber, Folate, Magnesium, Manganese, Potassium, Vitamin B6

White & Brown

- Cauliflower
- Garlic
- Onions
- Mushrooms
- Parsnips
- White Potatoes
- Apples
- Pears

- Chicory
- Cucumber

Key Nutrients: Anthoxanthins, Fiber, Folate, Magnesium Manganese, Potassium, Vitamin B6, Vitamin C, Vitamin K1

White fruits and vegetables have even been linked to lowering the risk of a stroke. In 2021, researchers at Wageningen University in The Netherlands found that a 25g a day increase in white fruits and vegetables were linked with a 9% lower risk of a stroke after examining 20,000 adults with an average age of 41 years old.

HEALTHY PROTEIN

As we mentioned in Chapter 7, protein is the building material that the body uses to construct every part of you. Protein is the fundamental building block of organs, muscle, skin and hormones. We need protein to help maintain and repair tissues (children need it for growth), send messages around the body, balance fluid levels, bolster immune health, and provide energy. There are more than 10,000 types of proteins in your body, and they are all made up of chains of amino acids. Out of the twenty amino acids that make up these proteins, nine cannot be made by the body. These are called essential amino acids and must be obtained from the foods we eat.

The UDS National Academy of Medicine recommends that adults consume a minimum of 0.8 g of protein for every kilogram of body weight. In other words, an individual weighing 70 kg (approximately 155 lb) would require 56 g of protein per day. However, protein intake can increase to up to 2 g per kilogram for more active individuals, depending on the activity. For example, a bodybuilder would consume a far higher protein content than a golfer. A diet that is high in protein may help to lower blood pressure, as well as fight conditions such as type 2 diabetes. Plus, protein helps you to stay fuller for longer, so can also help with appetite control.

The Best Protein Sources

While protein is a critical part of a healthy diet, many protein foods are high in calories and fat. It is important, therefore, that you make the right protein choices. Here are the ten top proteins that you should include on your plate:

1. White Fleshed Fish - white fish is extremely lean, with most varieties providing less than 3 grams of fat for a 100 g serving. That 100 g will also provide you with 20-25 g of protein. You should aim for two portions of fish per week.
2. Plain Greek Yogurt - a 170 g serving will provide 15-20 g of protein. Twice as much as you will get from regular yogurt!
3. Beans, Peas and Lentils - a 100 g serving of any of these legumes will average 8 g of protein and provide lots of fiber.
4. Skinless, white meat poultry - a 100 g serving of white meat chicken will provide 30 g of protein.

5. Low fat cottage cheese - a half cup of low-fat cottage cheese will provide 13 g of protein and just 2.5 g of fat.
6. Tofu - tofu is one of the very plant-based sources of all 11 essential amino acids. An 85 g serving will provide you with 7 g of protein.
7. Lean Beef - lean cuts of beef contain less than 10 g of fat. A 100 g lean cooked hamburger will provide you with 26 g of protein.
8. Low Fat Milk - A glass of 1% low-fat milk contains 8 g of protein and about 100 calories.
9. Eggs - an average-sized egg will provide 6 g of protein and 48 calories.
10. Pork Loin - pork tenderloin is the leanest cut of pork, providing 26 g of protein, 143 calories and 3.5 g of fat for every 100 g serving.

HEALTHY OILS

Healthy oils – suggested as an added extra by the Healthy Eating Plate – are a source of dietary fat. Dietary fat is a vital component of a healthy, balanced nutrition plan. There is a common belief that saturated fats are bad and unsaturated fats are good. However, good health requires a balance of fatty acids, including saturated fats. As saturated fats primarily come from animal sources, your quota of these will come from your 'Healthy Protein' section of the food plate. A good rule of thumb when it comes to saturated fat is that:

- Men should have no more than 30 grams of saturated fat daily
- Women should have no more than 20 grams of saturated fat daily

The majority of unsaturated fats, on the other hand, come from vegetable and plant sources. They come under two subcategories:

- Monounsaturated fats
- Polyunsaturated fats

Monounsaturated fats have the ability to reduce blood cholesterol levels and insulin levels. The best food sources of monounsaturated fats to include on your food plate are:

- Olives and olive oil
- Nuts and nut oils (e.g. coconut oil, peanut oil)
- Avocado
- Canola Oil

Unsaturated fats are also present in some types of fish, and are known as **omega-3 fatty acids**. Omega-3 fatty acids and other nutrients in fish may benefit heart health and reduce the risk of dying of heart disease. One of your recommended two portions of fish per week should be oily fish.

A good rule of thumb to follow when selecting healthy oils and fats is to avoid foods that are highly processed and that contain ingredients that you cannot even pronounce. Foods such as French Fries (and other deep-fried foods), crackers and baked goods are examples of foods that contain what are known as trans-fats. These fats are modified through the process of hydrogenation to preserve shelf life.

GUIDELINES ON SUGAR AND SALT

Finally, we need to talk about salt (sodium) and sugar.

High levels of sodium in the blood can contribute to inflammation. Over time, this can put you at serious risk of health issues such as high blood pressure, stroke, heart and kidney failure, and some cancers.

Despite this, salt is an important nutrient for the human body, so it is important that you don't cut it out completely! Instead, adults should aim to eat no more than 6 g of salt daily.

Consuming too much sugar, on the other hand, can lead to obesity, which itself is a risk factor for diabetes and heart disease. Excessive sugar in the diet can also lead to tooth decay. Current guidelines state that:

- No more than 5 percent of daily calories should come from sugar.
- Adults should have no more than 30 g of sugar

daily (7 sugar cubes).

EATING IN MODERATION

There is no such thing as good or bad food. There are most definitely foods that you should eat more often than others. Those are the ones that I've highlighted in the preceding sections. That doesn't mean that foods that are not on those lists are forbidden. Instead, they should be enjoyed occasionally. You will actually find when you limit them to occasional or treat time snacks, you will enjoy them a whole lot more.

Here are a dozen foods you should eat in moderation:

- French Fries
- Burgers
- Donuts
- Pizza
- Biscuits
- Ice Cream
- Alcohol
- Chocolate
- Snack Bars
- Potato Chips

RECAP OF KEY RECOMMENDATIONS:

1. The majority of your plate should be made up of plants. Eat at least 30 portions of a variety of

plant-based foods (wholegrains, fruit and vegetables) every week.
2. Eat lots of beans, pulses, fish, eggs, meat and other proteins (including 2 portions of fish every week, one of which should be oily).
3. Drink 6-8 cups/glasses of fluid a day, avoiding sugary drinks and alcohol. You will need more water if you exercise.
4. Foods high in saturated and/ or trans-fats, salt and sugar should be consumed in small amounts infrequently (no more than 6 g of salt, and 30 g of sugar on a daily basis).

PORTION SIZES

When it comes to how much food to actually fit on your plate per meal, it really does depend on a number of factors such as age, metabolism and physical activity. We're all different shapes and sizes and men and women have different recommended calorie intakes per day. Some of us prefer a bigger breakfast and a small dinner and vice versa.

We've already learned that smaller 9-inch plates and avoiding seconds will help reduce portion sizes but let's now look at dividing our daily calories up into meals, drinks and snacks. It's generally advised to eat your larger meals earlier in the day, so we'll go on that premise.

A woman's daily calorie intake in 2000, so let's break that down.

- Breakfast is 500 calories
- Lunch is 500 calories
- Dinner is 400 calories
- 400ml glass of 2% fat milk is 200 calories
- Snack number 1 is 200 calories.
- Snack number 2 is 200 calories
- 8 glasses of water is zero calories

A man's daily calorie intake is 2500, so as a man, you simply have an extra 500 calories per day to play around with.

This is just an example but I wouldn't recommend obsessing about calories, just as I do not recommend obsessing about the bathroom scales. There is give or take and you might need to eat more if you have been doing heavy resistance training or intense cardio that day. Keeping track of your calories is important but remember the key here is to follow the guidance in chapters 5 and 6, be mindful about your food, listen to your body and know when you are full.

SUMMARY

From this chapter, we really start to gain practical knowledge of what types of food we should eat. We can now start to proportion our meals in terms of macronutrients, knowing what our daily plate should look like. We also have vital micronutrient information to hand in order to put into practice and to go out to the grocery store and fill your fridge and pantry with color and diversity. As you can see there are dozens of fruits and vegetables that you can choose from. Be bold and experimental with your choices as only positive health benefits will come from a wide range of micronutrients. In our next chapter, we'll delve into a whole load of food tips as well as recipes for each daily meal to help get you started on your new and healthy lifestyle. We're almost there, so let's keep going!

9

CHANGES TO MAKE IN MEALS, SNACKS AND DESSERTS

"Food may be essential as fuel for the body, but GOOD food is fuel for the soul"

— MALCOLM FORBES

In our penultimate chapter, I reveal a range of simple ideas, suggestions and recipes that you can make immediately to improve your nutrition and improve your health. I'll divide them into sections based on the traditional three main meals of the day.

BREAKFAST

Here are ten tips to make every-day breakfasts healthier:

- Replace bacon rashes with medallions or turkey bacon. Or just one rash of regular bacon. Avoid streaky bacon as it is higher in fat.
- If you love sausages like most people do, cut down to just one sausage, find low-fat lean pork sausages, or use chicken or veggie ones.
- Try cauliflower hash browns instead of potato.
- Poach your eggs or use extra egg whites in your scrambled eggs or omelet for extra protein—no more than two yolks per person.
- Use semi skimmed or skimmed milk for oatmeal/porridge. There are also other great alternatives such as oat and almond milk.
- Change to wholemeal bread instead of white.
- Add in some vegetables or fruit. For example: grilled tomato, asparagus and tender stem broccoli are amazing with poached eggs.
- Add walnuts and a sprinkling of cinnamon to oatmeal.
- Include protein in the form of Greek yogurt.
- Blend up a breakfast smoothie, combining fruit, juice, yogurt, wheat germ, tofu and berries.

5 GREAT BREAKFAST RECIPE IDEAS

Banana Pancakes

Dry Ingredients

- 1.5 cups white whole wheat flour

- 1.5 teaspoons baking powder
- 1/2 teaspoon ground cinnamon
- 1/8 teaspoon salt

Wet Ingredients

- 2 medium bananas, mashed (~1 cup puree)
- 2 large eggs
- 1 teaspoon vanilla extract
- 1 cup unsweetened almond milk
- 3 tablespoons melted coconut oil
- Drizzle of honey (optional)

Method

1. First, combine dry ingredients in a medium bowl and set aside.
2. Mash bananas in a large bowl until there are only a few lumps and they are pureed. Then, add in eggs, vanilla, and almond milk and whisk until smooth.
3. Slowly add dry ingredients to wet and mix to combine. Finally, add in melted coconut oil and mix until smooth. Your batter should be thick.
4. Heat a non-stick pan over medium heat. Spray with coconut oil cooking spray. When the oil is hot, scoop about 1/3 cup of the batter onto your pan and cook for 2-3 minutes on each side, flipping when the bubbles start to form in the center of the pancakes.

5. Repeat until all batter is gone.
6. Top with sliced banana and honey.

Low Carb Breakfast Burritos

Ingredients

- 2 large eggs
- 1 tbsp. Skimmed milk
- 1 tbsp. Freshly chopped chives
- Sprinkle of salt
- Freshly ground black pepper
- 1 tbsp. Butter
- 2 slices cooked bacon
- 1/2 c. Black beans
- 1 avocado, thinly sliced
- 1/2 c. shredded cheddar
- Salsa, for serving

Method

1. In a small bowl, whisk together eggs, milk, and chives, and season with salt and pepper.
2. In a large non-stick skillet, melt butter. Once the pan is completely coated, add the egg mixture. Tilt pan back and forth to make sure it's completely coated, then let cook, 2 minutes. Once you can move the egg back and forth, carefully flip and cook 2 minutes more.
3. Transfer to a plate and top with bacon, black

beans, avocado, cheddar, and salsa. Roll up into a burrito and serve.

Smoked Salmon and Poached Egg with Green Vegetables

Ingredients

- 50g smoked salmon
- 2 medium eggs
- 4 sticks of asparagus
- 4 sticks tender stem broccoli
- 1/4 tsp. Salt
- 1/4 tsp. Black pepper
- 30-40 mg. White wine vinegar
- ¼ squeezed lemon

Method

1. Turn your grill to a medium-high heat and place the asparagus and broccoli under the grill for 5 minutes, turning half way.
2. Bring a saucepan of water and the white wine vinegar to medium heat so it's lightly bubbling.
3. Crack the 2 eggs and poach for 2 – 2 ½ minutes. Meanwhile, place the salmon on the plate.
4. Place the eggs on some kitchen paper to soak up any remaining water.
5. Serve eggs and vegetables on the plate. Squeeze the lemon and season according to taste.

Easy Kale Feta Egg Toast

Ingredients

- 2 slices English muffin bread, sourdough bread, multigrain bread, or English muffin, for serving
- 3 teaspoons olive oil divided
- 3 cups chopped kale stems removed
- 1 teaspoon minced garlic (2 cloves)
- 1/8 teaspoon salt plus additional for seasoning
- 1/8 teaspoon pepper plus additional for seasoning
- 1/8 teaspoon red pepper flakes
- 2 large eggs
- 2 ounces feta cheese crumbled

Method

1. Toast bread in a toaster, toaster oven, or beneath a broiler. Set aside.
2. Heat 2 teaspoons of olive oil in a large skillet on medium heat. Add the kale, stir to coat, then cook, occasionally stirring, until the kale begins to soften, about 5 minutes.
3. Add the garlic, ⅛ teaspoon salt, ⅛ teaspoon pepper, and red pepper flakes. Stir and cook for 1 additional minute. Remove from heat, stir in the feta cheese, then cover to keep warm.
4. In a small skillet, heat the remaining teaspoon of olive oil over medium. Gently crack eggs into

skillet and sprinkle with a little extra salt and pepper.
5. Cook until the whites are nearly set, about 1 minute. Cover skillet, remove from heat and let stand until whites are set but yolks are still soft, about 3 minutes.
6. To serve: Place half of the kale on top of each toast, then top with a fried egg. Serve immediately.

Frittatas

Ingredients

- ¼ c. Spinach
- ¼ c. Chopped onion
- ¼ c. Chopped peppers
- 1 tomato sliced
- 2 eggs
- ¼ c. Crumbled feta
- Salt and pepper to season
- 1 tbsp. Olive oil
- 2 slices of wholemeal toast
- Watercress

Method

1. Wisk the 2 eggs in a bowl with a splash of milk if desired and add salt and pepper to taste. Chop the tomato into thin slices.

2. Heat the olive oil in a frying pan on a medium-high heat and heat your grill to a high temperature.
3. Add the onions and peppers to the pan for 3 minutes then the spinach for 1 more minute.
4. Add the eggs and make sure they cover the whole frying pan.
5. Place the tomato slices on top and sprinkle the feta.
6. Put toast on in the toaster and heat the frittata on the pan for 2 minutes on a medium heat.
7. Place the frying pan under the grill for 2 minutes.
8. Butter the toast, place the water cress on the side.
9. Fold the Frittata in half if desired and serve.

5 GREAT LUNCH IDEAS

Easy Healthy Salad Sandwich

Ingredients

For the herb mayo

- 1/3 cup mayonnaise
- ¼ cup fresh herbs of your choice (basil, parsley, chives)
- a squeeze of lemon juice
- salt and pepper to taste

For the sandwich

- 2 slices whole-grain bread
- sliced tomato
- sliced cucumber
- sliced red onion
- julienned carrot
- lettuce / arugula / baby spinach
- sliced cheese (optional)

Method

1. Combine all the mayo ingredients and blend with an immersion blender until smooth. Alternatively, use a blender or food processor.
2. To assemble the sandwich, spread a generous dollop of the mayo onto each slice of bread and top with the vegetables and cheese. Sandwich, slice and serve.

Spiced Lentil & Butternut Squash Soup

Ingredients

- 2 tbsp olive oil
- 2 onions, finely chopped
- 2 garlic cloves, crushed
- ¼ tsp hot chili powder
- 1 tbsp ras el hanout
- 1 butternut squash, peeled and cut into 2cm pieces
- 100g red lentils
- 1liter hot vegetable stock

- 1 small bunch coriander, leaves chopped, plus extra to serve
- Natural yogurt, to serve

Method

1. Heat the oil in a large flameproof casserole dish or saucepan over medium-high heat. Fry the onions with a pinch of salt for 7 mins, or until softened and just caramelized. Add the garlic, chili and ras el hanout, and cook for 1 min more.
2. Stir in the squash and lentils. Pour over the stock and season to taste. Bring to the boil, then reduce the heat to a simmer and cook, cover for 25 mins or until the squash is soft.
3. Blitz the soup with a stick blender until smooth, then season to taste. To freeze, leave to cool completely and transfer to large freezer-proof bags.
4. Stir in the coriander leaves and ladle the soup into bowls. Serve topped with the dukkah, yogurt and extra coriander leaves.

Bright and Spicy Shrimp Noodle Salad

Ingredients

- ⅓ cup fresh lime juice
- 2 tsp. honey
- 1 serrano chile, very thinly sliced
- 1 inch piece of ginger, peeled, finely grated
- 1 garlic clove, finely grated
- 1 Tbsp plus 1½ tsp fish sauce
- 4 Tbsp. extra-virgin olive oil
- Salt
- 1 lb. large shrimp (preferably wild), peeled, deveined
- 6 oz. bean thread (cellophane or glass) noodles
- 1 cucumber, halved lengthwise, thinly sliced crosswise
- ½ cup salted, roasted peanuts, crushed
- 1 cup basil leaves

Method

1. Stir lime juice and honey in a small bowl until honey dissolves. Mix in chile, ginger, garlic, fish sauce, and 3 Tbsp of oil; season dressing with salt.
2. Toss shrimp and 2 Tbsp of dressing in a medium bowl to coat; let sit for 10 minutes.
3. Meanwhile, cook noodles according to package directions. Drain and add to the bowl with

remaining dressing along with cucumber and ¼ cup peanuts; toss well.
4. Heat remaining 1 Tbsp of oil in a large nonstick skillet over medium-high. Pour off any liquid from shrimp and pat dry; season all over with salt. Cook shrimp, occasionally tossing, until browned and bright pink, about 5 minutes. Transfer to a bowl with noodles, add basil and toss well to combine.
5. Divide noodle salad among bowls and top with remaining peanuts.

Lemony Salmon and Spiced Chickpeas

Ingredients

- 1 lemon, thinly sliced, seeds removed
- ½ cup extra-virgin olive oil, plus more for drizzling
- 1½-lb. salmon fillet, preferably skin-on
- ½ tsp. Salt
- Freshly ground black pepper
- 15-oz. can chickpeas, rinsed, patted dry
- 1 garlic clove, finely chopped
- 2 tsp. za'atar
- 1 tsp. fresh lemon juice
- 4 cups baby arugula or baby spinach
- 4 radishes, trimmed, thinly sliced
- Flaky sea salt

Method

1. Place a rack in the lower third of the oven; preheat to 300°. Toss lemon slices in a large bowl with a drizzle of oil. Arrange slices in an even layer on a rimmed baking sheet. Set salmon on lemons. Season salmon all over with salt and pepper, then drizzle and rub with some oil. Roast until the salmon is just barely opaque in the middle, 12–17 minutes, depending on thickness. If you like your salmon well-done, cook it a few minutes longer, but keep in mind that you risk the chance it will dry out. Let salmon cool, then flake into medium-size pieces with a fork.
2. Meanwhile, bring chickpeas, garlic, za'atar, and remaining ½ cup oil to a bare simmer in a small skillet over medium-low heat. Cook, stirring occasionally and reducing heat if needed, 10 minutes. Stir in ½ tsp of salt (less if your za'atar is salty) and remove skillet from heat.
3. Using a slotted spoon, transfer chickpeas to a medium bowl, leaving oil behind. Whisk lemon juice into oil; taste dressing and season with more salt and a few grinds of pepper if needed.
4. Toss arugula in a large bowl with 1 tsp of dressing. Divide among bowls along with radishes, chickpeas, and salmon (and lemons if desired); drizzle with more dressing. Sprinkle it with sea salt and more pepper.

Bean Salad Bowl with Asian Glaze

Ingredients

For the salad

- Broad beans
- Green beans
- Red onion
- Cherry tomatoes
- Cucumber
- Mixed peppers
- Leafy greens like spinach, rocket, watercress or lettuce
- Quinoa
- Pre-cooked shrimp, sliced chicken or steak (optional)

For the Asian glaze (serves 4, so save some in the fridge for another meal)

- 3 cloves chopped garlic
- 1 inch block of ginger, chopped
- ¼ cup. honey
- ¼ cup of soy sauce
- 3 tablespoons of rice vinegar
- 2 tablespoons hoisin sauce
- 1 tablespoon sesame oil
- ½ teaspoon of chilli flakes (optional for spice)

Method

1. Lightly boil the broad and green beans for 3 minutes, then run them under cold water
2. In a pan, lightly boil the quinoa, usually about 15 mins (check the packaging for cooking time)
3. Chop the onion, tomato and cucumber
4. If desired, grill your chicken breast or steak of choice, then cut into slices. Let it cool down
5. Add the sauce ingredients into a pan and gently boil for 5 minutes. Keep stirring to avoid it sticking to the pan. Let it cool down
6. Add the leafy greens, beans and all other veg into a bowl
7. Once the quinoa is done, let it cool down and add to the bowl
8. Add your chicken, steak or pre-cooked cold shrimp on top, then add the glaze

DINNER

My Top 22 Tips

1. Make a roast chicken for dinner, use the remaining meat for chicken salads and sandwiches, and boil the bones to make stock for healthy soups.
2. Use turkey thigh or breast mince (thigh is much tastier) instead of red meat mince like beef or lamb.
3. Make mash from either sweet potato or cannellini beans rather than white potato.

4. If you hate broccoli, try grilled or pan-fried tender stem broccoli to help introduce you to the flavor.
5. Use seasonings, herbs and spices for your meat and fish rather than sauces.
6. Use things like lemon, lime, wine, olive oils for lighter dressings rather than creamy sauces.
7. Use crème fresh instead of cream for sauces and desserts.
8. Find a low sugar protein bar with fiber that you really like or better yet make your own, and always have one on you as a healthier snack instead of a candy bar.
9. Use Greek yogurt (full fat) with a drizzle of honey and fruit rather than store-bought yogurt or unhealthy desserts.
10. Freeze your bread so you don't need to rush using it before the use-by date.
11. Buy a juicer and make your own fresh fruit juice instead of added sugar fruit juice from the shops.
12. Buy a Nutribullet and make your own fruit and veg smoothies or protein shakes. Add whole oats for extra fiber.
13. Learn to poach an egg as it's quick and healthy.
14. If you're craving something fizzy, drink sparkling mineral water with no added sugar squash instead of high sugary sodas.
15. Half and half Courgette aka Zucchini with pasta to avoid meals like bolognaise or carbonara being too high in carb.

16. Try to get used to brown rice and pasta over time. Brown basmati is nicer, so start with that.
17. Instead of salted crisps as snacks, eat nuts. Unsalted almonds, walnuts, brazil and cashew are high in nutrition.
18. When making stir fry meals, use it as an opportunity to add in as much vegetables as possible. Buy a good stir fry veg mix, add in green beans, sugar snap peas, broccoli, spring greens… the list goes on and on! Mix up your meat or fish, i.e. One week pork, the next week shrimp, the next week vegetables only!
19. Try to avoid using packaged stir fry sauces and make your own. Personally, ginger, chilli, lemon and lime juice, a splash of soy sauce, and a splash of white wine work great!
20. Replace the frying pan with your grill or an air fryer. For example, Grilled bacon, pork chops, chicken etc. You can boil your potatoes then put them in the air fryer for 5-10 minutes and they will crispen up without using all that oil in a frying pan. This also works well with steak!
21. If you hate or simply don't have time to always chop up vegetables, buy frozen chopped vegetables like onions and peppers to save time and stress.
22. Cook healthy bulk meals and portion them up straight away into Tupperware so you have extra meals for lunches or dinners. This will also prevent you from having seconds after dinner.

5 GREAT DINNER IDEAS

Spanish Chicken

Ingredients

- 4 boneless skinless chicken breasts - OR 6 chicken thighs
- 3 tablespoons vegetable or canola oil
- 1 cup uncooked brown basmati rice
- 2 ¼ cups low salt chicken broth
- 1 lemon
- chopped cilantro or parsley - for garnish
- Green vegetables like broccoli, sugar snap peas, spring greens

For the Spanish Mix Seasoning

- 2 teaspoons smoked paprika
- 1 teaspoon garlic powder
- 1 teaspoon salt
- 1 teaspoon ground cumin
- 1 teaspoon chili powder
- 1 teaspoon coriander
- ¼ teaspoon Italian seasoning

Method

1. In a small bowl, whisk together all ingredients for the Spanish seasoning mix. Divide in half and set aside. Cut the lemon in half, then thinly slice one half - for garnish - and reserve the other half for juicing later in the recipe.
2. Place chicken in a medium bowl. Drizzle with 2 tablespoons of oil, then toss to coat well. Use half of the prepared seasoning mix to rub on both sides of each piece of chicken.
3. Drizzle a large skillet with the remaining 1 tablespoon of oil and bring to medium heat. Cook chicken for 2-3 minutes on each side until browned. Transfer to a plate. (It won't be cooked through at this point).
4. Add rice, chicken broth, juice from 1/2 of the lemon, and remaining seasoning mix and stir to combine. Return the chicken to the pan on top of the rice. Cover and cook for 20-25 minutes until liquid is absorbed, rice is tender, and chicken is cooked through.
5. Steam the extra vegetables of choice according to the packet guidelines.
6. Garnish with lemon slices and freshly chopped cilantro or parsley and serve immediately.

Turkey Mince Bolognaise with Zucchini and Extra Vegetables

Ingredients

- 500g turkey thigh mince
- Half an onion
- 1 green pepper
- 1 large carrot
- 1 stick of celery
- 1 zucchini aka courgette
- 1 ½ tins chopped tomato
- 1 small lemon (juice)
- Italian herbs
- Fresh basil
- 1 beef stockpot
- 3 cloves of garlic
- Salt and pepper
- Olive oil
- Splash of red wine
- Wholemeal spaghetti
- A light sprinkle of grated cheese (if desired)

Method

1. Chop the onions, peppers, carrots and celery into small pieces.
2. Heat the oil in a large pan or wok on a medium-high heat.
3. Add the onions, peppers, carrots and celery into the pan and fry for 2-3 minutes.
4. Add the mince and cook till brown. Meanwhile, chop the garlic into small pieces.

5. Boil the water for the pasta and add a pinch of salt.
6. Add the tomatoes, wine, lemon juice, Italian herbs, stockpot, salt, pepper and garlic into the pan and simmer on a medium heat for 20 minutes.
7. Cook the pasta on the hob for 8-10 minutes.
8. If you have a spiralizer, prepare the zucchini. You do not need to cook the zucchini. Place the spaghetti and zucchini into a bowl (half and half), then the sauce on top.
9. Grate the cheese and place the fresh basil on top.

Shrimp & Broccoli

Ingredients

- 1 pound large shrimp, deveined (peeled or unpeeled)
- 1 1/2 pounds broccoli (heads and stems)
- 1 small white onion
- 2 tablespoons rice vinegar
- 4 tablespoons soy sauce
- ½ tablespoon chili garlic sauce (optional)
- 2 tablespoons sesame oil
- ¼ teaspoon salt
- Sesame seeds, for garnish
- Thinly sliced green onion for garnish (optional)
- To serve: rice or noodles

Method

1. If frozen, thaw the shrimp according to the package instructions or the notes above.
2. Chop the broccoli into small bite-sized pieces. Cut the onion into wide slices.
3. In a measuring cup, stir together the rice vinegar, soy sauce, and chili garlic sauce.
4. If serving with rice, remember to allow time for the rice to cook. Usually around 10 minutes for white and 20 - 25 minutes for brown. If serving with noodles, usually allow 3- 5 minutes. Check all packaging first to get your timing right.
5. In a large skillet or wok, heat the sesame oil over medium-high heat. Add the broccoli, onion and salt and cook for 5 to 6 minutes until fork-tender, stirring occasionally. Add the shrimp and cook for 3 to 4 minutes, stirring frequently.
6. When the shrimp is just about opaque, add the sauce mixture and cook for 1 minute. Remove from the heat. Serve with sesame seeds.

Grilled Chicken with Charred Pineapple Salad

Ingredients

- 1 teaspoon dried oregano
- Olive oil
- 2 x 150 g free-range chicken breasts
- 150 g quinoa
- 50 g white cabbage
- 1 large handful of salad leaves

- ¼ of a pineapple
- 50 g natural Greek yogurt
- 1 fresh red chili

Dressing

- ½ an avocado
- ½ a bunch of fresh coriander, (15g)
- 2 tablespoons pickled jalapeños
- 2 limes

Method

1. Combine the oregano in a bowl with 1 to 2 tablespoons of oil, then season with sea salt and black pepper.
2. Use a sharp knife to slice into the chicken breasts, then open each one out flat like a book to butterfly. Place in the bowl with the herby oil, turning until well coated, then leave to one side.
3. Cook the quinoa according to the packet instructions, then drain and set aside.
4. For the dressing, peel and destone the avocado half, then scoop the flesh into a blender. Add half the coriander (stalks and all) and the jalapeños, along with a splash of the pickling liquid and the juice of 1½ limes. Blitz until smooth, adding a splash of oil if needed. Stir through the quinoa.
5. Finely shred the cabbage, pick the remaining coriander leaves, then toss with the salad leaves.
6. Place a griddle pan over high heat. Peel the pineapple, remove and discard any core, then chop into 4. Place on the hot griddle pan for a few minutes on each side, or until charred, and transfer to a chopping board. In the same pan, griddle the chicken for 5 minutes on each side, or until charred and cooked through, then remove from the pan and leave to rest on the board for a few minutes.
7. Chop the griddled pineapple into bite-sized

chunks, then slice the chicken into thin strips. Deseed and finely chop the chili.

8. Divide the yogurt between four plates, then top with the chicken, adding the pineapple on one side and the dressed quinoa on the other. Toss the leaves and cabbage with the juice of the remaining lime half and a little salt and pepper, plus the chopped chili. Divide between the plates, then serve.

Steak Dijon

Ingredients

- 4 medium sweet potatoes
- 2 steaks of choice
- 1 tbsp. canola oil
- 1 medium onion
- 1 c. low salt chicken broth
- 2 tbsp. finely chopped fresh dill
- 1 tbsp. Dijon mustard
- 1 lb. green beans

Method

1. Peel the Sweet potatoes then, in a pan of boiling water, carefully add the potatoes and slow boil them on medium-high heat until soft. Drain well.
2. Meanwhile, in a 12-inch skillet, heat oil on medium-high. Sprinkle steaks with 1/4 teaspoon each salt and pepper; cook 2 to 3 minutes per side on medium-high heat or until the desired doneness. Transfer to a cutting board and cover with foil.
3. In the same skillet, cook the onion for 2 minutes, stirring. Stir in broth; heat to simmering. Simmer for 5 minutes. Whisk in dill, mustard, and 1/4 teaspoon pepper.
4. Steam the green beans as directed on the packet. Usually 3-4 minutes.
5. Mash sweet potatoes. You will not need any butter, milk, cheese or salt.
6. Slice steak; serve with potatoes, green beans, and sauce.

10 HEALTHIER DESSERT OPTIONS

1. Fruit
2. Chia Pudding
3. Greek Yogurt
4. Peanut Butter and Banana Ice Cream
5. Low Sugar Popsicles

6. Nut Butter
7. Baked Pears or Apples
8. Chocolate Dipped Banana Bites
9. DIY Chocolate Truffles
10. Baked Sweet Potatoes

MAKE YOUR OWN PROTEIN BARS

Protein bars provide a convenient on-the-go protein source. However, store-bought bars are both expensive and liable to contain fillers, flavorings and preservatives. You can and should make your own no-bake protein bars.

Protein Nut Bar Recipe

Ingredients

- 2 1/2 cups (250 g) old-fashioned certified gluten-free rolled oats (if gluten-free isn't necessary, use any oats)
- 1 1/2 scoops (54 g) gluten-free protein powder (I like Vega essentials chocolate flavor protein powder, but you can use whey protein or your favorite protein powder (vanilla or chocolate))
- 1/2 cup (40 g) unsweetened cocoa powder (natural or Dutch-processed) (can replace with more protein powder)
- 3/4 cup (192 g) smooth natural nut butter (I have used peanut butter, almond butter and cashew butter—all work well)
- 1/4 cup (84 g) pure maple syrup

- 1/4 teaspoon salt
- 1/4 cup (2 fluid ounces) milk (any kind), plus more as necessary
- 3 ounces unsweetened chocolate, chopped and melted (can replace with 2 tablespoons more nut butter + 1 tablespoon pure maple syrup)
- 8 ounces bittersweet chocolate, chopped and melted (optional, for coating)

Method

1. Line an 8-inch square baking pan or standard 9-inch x 5-inch loaf pan with unbleached parchment paper and set it aside.
2. To make the date version, place the oats in a food processor fitted with the steel blade and process until ground into flour. Add the protein powder, dates, maple syrup, vanilla, salt, 1/4 cup milk and (optional) melted unsweetened chocolate. Process until the mixture is well-combined and is tacky (but not sticky) to the touch. Add more milk by the teaspoonful and process, only as necessary for the mixture to reach the proper consistency. If you opt not to use the melted unsweetened chocolate, you will have to add more milk, and the bars will not hold together as firmly when shaped.
3. Transfer the mixture to the prepared pan and press firmly into an even layer, smoothing the top as much as possible. Cover with parchment and place in the refrigerator or freezer to chill until

firm (about 1 hour in the refrigerator, or 20 minutes in the freezer). Remove the bars from the pan and slice them into 10 or 12 equal-sized rectangular bars. Dip in the optional melted bittersweet chocolate to coat and allow to sit at room temperature until set. Store the bars in a sealed container in the refrigerator.

4. To make the nut butter version, place the oats in a food processor fitted with the steel blade and process until ground into flour. Add the protein powder, cocoa powder (or more protein powder), nut butter, maple syrup, salt, 1/4 cup milk and melted unsweetened chocolate (or more nut butter and maple syrup). Process until the mixture is well-combined and is tacky (but not sticky) to the touch. Add more milk by the teaspoonful and process, only as necessary for the mixture to reach the proper consistency.

5. Transfer the mixture to the prepared pan and press firmly into an even layer, smoothing the top as much as possible. Cover with parchment and place in the refrigerator or freezer to chill until firm (about 1 hour in the refrigerator, or 20 minutes in the freezer). Remove the bars from the pan and slice into 10 or 12 equal-sized rectangular bars. Dip in the optional melted bittersweet chocolate to coat or simply drizzle some melted chocolate over the top, and allow to sit at room temperature until set. Wrap the bars individually in waxed paper, and store in the refrigerator.

THE SMOOTHIE SOLUTION

Getting into the Smoothie habit will make it a whole lot easier for you to provide your body with the nutrients it needs to thrive.

Here are 5 reasons why you should embrace the smoothie habit...

Lowered Cholesterol

High levels of low-density lipoprotein (LDL) cholesterol have been associated with all manner of cardiac problems. Getting into the smoothie habit will help to lower your LDL cholesterol levels. If you replace a breakfast of bacon, eggs and toast with a fruit-filled smoothie, you will automatically cut back your LDL cholesterol intake. On top of that, the fruits that are included in your smoothies are filled with phytochemicals, antioxidants and other properties that reduce LDL cholesterol. The best fruits to include to bring down your LDL cholesterol levels are apples, blueberries, strawberries, avocados, grapes and citrus fruits.

Immunity-Boosting

The vitamins, minerals, phytochemicals and antioxidants that are in smoothies will boost your immunity. This will better ward off colds, flu and viruses. Focus on citrus juices to get the most immunity-boosting benefit from your smoothies.

Heart Health

We have already mentioned how smoothies can help lower LDL cholesterol levels. But that's not the only way they benefit your heart health. Including citrus fruits in your smoothies will provide you with potassium and folate. Potassium helps to keep your blood pressure levels in check, while folate helps to produce healthy blood cells.

Improves Digestion

When you drink a fruit-infused smoothie, you will be taking in between 2 and 7 grams of fiber. This will help to keep your digestive system functioning with maximum efficiency. When you take your fruits in the form of a smoothie, the process of digestion is much easier because the fruits are already partially broken down. This helps to eliminate such digestive problems as gas, bloating and indigestion that many people experience when they eat fruit.

Convenience

Let's face it – our lives are busy. Finding the time to prepare a proper dinner meal is challenging enough. Preparing several nutritionally balanced meals over the course of your day can be totally overwhelming. But when you replace one of those meals with a super delicious, quick-to-prepare smoothie, suddenly things become way more manageable.

3 GREAT SMOOTHIE RECIPES

Berry Explosion

Ingredients

- 1 x Scoop of Strawberry Protein Powder
- 1/2 cup of Blueberries
- ½ cup of raspberries
- 4 strawberries
- 1 x Cup of Coconut Milk
- 2-3 Ice Cubes

Method

1. Place the berries in your blender
2. Add 1 cup of unsweetened Coconut Milk
3. Add 2-3 Ice cubes
4. Add the Strawberry Protein Powder
5. Blend all ingredients for 30-45 sec

Green Power Cleansing Juice

Ingredients

- 2 x Big kale leaves
- 1/2 Cup x baby spinach leaves
- 1 x chopped cucumber
- 1 x apple roughly chopped
- 1 x Lemon peeled
- 1/2 Bunch mint

- Option to add ginger

Method

1. Juice all ingredients together in a juicer and pour over ice if desired.

Tropical Protein Heaven

Ingredients

1. 1 x cup coconut milk
2. 1/2 x banana
3. 1/2 cup x chopped pineapple
4. 1/2 cup x chopped mango
5. 2 scoops x Vanilla Protein Powder
6. crushed ice

Method

1. Blend all ingredients and pour over ice.

Many recipes in this chapter are courtesy of:

www.wellplated.com
www.feastingathome.com
www.acouplecooks.com
www.jamieoliver.com
www.delish.com
https://glutenfreeonashoestring.com
https://www.modernhoney.com
https://drivemehungry.com/sweet-and-tangy-sticky-soy-glaze/

SUMMARY

There are literally millions of food ideas, tips and recipes out there. We all have different tastes and dietary requirements, some of which require very specific attention to detail. For most of you reading this chapter, you will be able to take the majority of these recipes and put them into practice. This is also a great opportunity to expand your food knowledge as there's a whole new world out there of amazing chefs and recipe books. You could even take it a step further and sign up to either weekly cooking classes or a one-off weekend masterclass. The options are all out there for you so take advantage of them! Remember, food is a gift. It's meant to be appreciated, respected but most importantly embraced and enjoyed!

CONCLUSION

"Success is not final. Failure is not fatal. It is the courage to continue that counts"

— SIR WINSTON CHURCHILL

Over the course of our journey together, we have charted a course toward new, better, healthier eating habits that you can easily adopt and ingrain into your lifestyle. In the process, you have discovered how to finally break the bad habits that have been enslaving you to a way of eating that you've known is no good but been powerless to do anything about. Well, now you have the power!

How have we done it?

At the outset, I laid out our template for success. It was based on the following 3 fundamental steps:

Step 1 – Identifying habits throughout our lives and understanding why these have manifested.

Step 2 – Change our mindset and learn how to break those habits through self-reflection, honesty and mindful eating techniques.

Step 3 – Implement practical knowledge solutions to provide you with a detailed basic education in nutrition, along with valuable tips and meal ideas.

Let's now review the key takeaways under each of these steps...

STEP ONE: IDENTIFYING HABITS

During our formative years, we develop the habits that will drive your nutritional future. The habits are a combination of prenatal nutrition, cultural differences, food company advertising, parental example, social media influences, peer pressure, and societal pressures.

What We've Learnt About Ourselves

1. Ageing. As we age, our bodies undergo the following detrimental changes...

- We get fatter
- Allergies become more of an issue
- Plaque builds up on our arteries

- We sweat less
- We reduce muscle mass
- The brain shrinks
- Our teeth become less sensitive
- Our skin becomes thinner, less elastic and drier
- Our hair becomes less vibrant
- We get shorter
- The bladder becomes weaker
- Our heart activity slows down
- Our taste sensation is reduced
- Our hormonal activity changes
- Our bone density decreases
- We experience digestive system disorders

To offset these changes, we need to adjust how we eat. The key change is to reduce daily caloric intake, with a focus on vegetables, fruits, lean meats and fish.

2. Stress. Stress has a direct impact on our physical health, especially digestion and gut health. The best nutrients to reduce stress are:

- Potassium
- B Vitamins
- Calcium
- Omega-3 Fatty Acids
- Iodine

3. Dieting. Dieting is not the solution to long-term weight loss. When you go on a diet, the following things occur . . .

- Your metabolism slows down
- Your body kicks into fight or flight mode
- Your cortisol levels increase
- Stress levels rise
- You fixate on forbidden foods
- You tend to lose muscle tissue, water and minerals over fat

STEP TWO: CHANGING MINDSET

A powerful impetus to breaking free from the eating rules that enslave us is the concept of mindfulness. Mindful eating involves:

- Controlling what comes into the house
- Not allowing yourself to get too hungry
- Buying smaller plates
- Savoring your food
- Engaging all your senses
- Chewing your food thoroughly
- Slowing down

The two key hormones that regulate hunger are...

- Leptin
- Ghrelin

In order to balance these key hormones, you need to:

- Get 7-8 hours of sleep each night

- Eat protein with every meal
- Do regular exercise. High-Intensity Interval Training (HIIT) Workouts are ideal
- Eat more high fiber foods

The three parts of the Habit Loop are ...

- The Trigger
- The Behaviour
- The Reward

Remember, switching from a bad habit to a good habit doesn't have to require changing all three of these steps. If you stick with the same trigger and reward but simply switch out the action in the middle, you will be able to transform a bad habit into a good habit.

STEP 3: PRACTICAL SOLUTIONS

In Chapters 8 and 9, you were presented with dozens of practical tips, food recommendations and recipes to kickstart your nutritional transformation and establish your new, healthy nutritional habits. Some of these included:

Balance

You need to balance all 3 macronutrients in your nutritional plan. Carbohydrates, which provide glucose, are the most efficient energy source. Carbs also provide fiber, which promotes satiety and boosts gut health. Good health requires a balance of fatty acids, including saturated fats. Fats, in the form of triglycerides, are the major form of fat storage in the body. Protein, in the form of amino acids, makes up the building material of the body.

The Harvard Healthy Eating plate represents a good eating plan to follow. The key recommendations are . . .

- Fruits and vegetables: ½ plate
- Whole grains: ¼ plate
- Protein: ¼ plate
- Healthy plant oils: in moderation

Hydration

Water is essential to the efficient functioning of the body. Aim to drink 8 glasses of water each day. Sleep is also crucial to overall health, being especially important for renewing energy levels and relieving stress.

Recommended Maximum Daily Intakes

- Men should have no more than 30 grams of saturated fat daily.
- Women should have no more than 20 grams of saturated fat daily.
- No more than 5 percent of daily calories should come from sugar.
- Adults should have no more than 30 grams of sugar daily (7 sugar cubes).
- Adults should eat no more than 6 grams of salt daily.

Other Top Tips

- Add color to your plate by choosing vegetables that cover the rainbow. Eat at least 5 portions of a variety of fruit and vegetables every day. 2 fruit and 3 vegetable ideally.
- Do not classify food as good and bad. Instead, separate them as either frequent or occasional selections.
- Eat some dairy or dairy alternatives (such as oat

drinks); choosing lower fat and lower sugar options.
- Eat beans, pulses, fish, eggs, meat and other proteins (including 2 portions of fish every week, one of which should be oily).
- Avoid processed spreads like margarine and eat natural butter in small amounts.
- Foods high in fat, salt and sugar should be consumed in small amounts infrequently.

By putting all of this into practice, you'll no longer have to feel like a driver at the wheel of a runaway car. Those bad eating habits that you've been enslaved to for as long as you can remember will be things of the past, and you will be free to move forward with your new, better eating habits. Then you'll be able to wake up every day feeling that you are living inside of a well-maintained, tight machine that not only looks good but is functioning at its best. At the same time, you will have developed a new appreciation for food, relishing its nourishing properties and delighting in the abundance of exquisite flavor and variety.

You now have the power, so go and put it to use!

> "Success isn't always about greatness. It's about consistency. Consistent hard work gains success. Greatness will come"
>
> — DWAYNE JOHNSON

Thank you for purchasing 'Total Fitness and Nutrition After 40: 2-in-1 Value Bundle'
If you have enjoyed this book, please leave a review on Amazon.

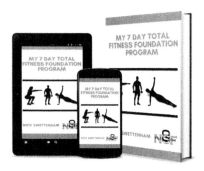

A Special Gift For My Readers

Included with the purchase of this book is My 7 Day Total Fitness Foundation Program to help you get started on your fitness journey. This program is a great way to start or adapt your training using all my 7 foundations. Click the link below and let us know which email address you would like it delivered to.

www.nickswettenhamfitness.com

REFERENCES

CHAPTER 1

https://www.sciencedaily.com/releases/2008/06/080630200951.htm#:~:text=FULL%20STORY-,Mothers%20who%20eat%20an%20unhealthy%20diet%20during%20pregnancy%20may%20be,to%20new%20research(1)

CHAPTER 2

Age-related decline in RMR in physically active men: relation to exercise volume and energy intake - v) PubMed (nih.go

https://pubmed.ncbi.nlm.nih.gov/18175749/

https://academic.oup.com/advances/article/3/1/54/4644546

https://agsjournals.onlinelibrary.wiley.com/doi/full/10.1111/j.1532-5415.2008.01732.x

Serum Lutein is related to Relational Memory Performance - PubMed (nih.gov)

Health benefits of anthocyanins and molecular mechanisms: Update from recent decade - PubMed (nih.gov)

Effect of a 12-Week Almond-Enriched Diet on Biomarkers of Cognitive Performance, Mood, and Cardiometabolic Health in Older Overweight Adults - PubMed (nih.gov)

CHAPTER 3

https://psychologyofeating.com/the-stress-metabolism-connection/

https://barbend.com/stress-strength-training/

https://www.healthline.com/health/stress/effects-on-body#4

https://www.healthline.com/health/cortisol-urine

Cholesterol in Eggs May Not Hurt Heart Health: Study – WebMD

https://www.hindawi.com/journals/jobe/2011/651936/

https://www.ucsf.edu/news/2004/11/5230/ucsf-led-study-suggests-link-between-psychological-stress-and-cell-aging

https://www.mayoclinic.org/healthy-lifestyle/stress-management/in-depth/art-20046037

https://www.ncbi.nlm.nih.gov/pmc/articles/PMC3181836/

https://www.livestrong.com/article/460992-does-stress-increase-metabolism/

https://www.jneurosci.org/content/33/17/7234

CHAPTER 4

R. Cleland et al., "Commercial Weight Loss Products and Programs: What Consumers Stand to Gain and Lose. A Public Conference on the Information Consumers Need to Evaluate Weight Loss Products and Programs," Critical Reviews in Food Science and Nutrition 41, no. 1 (January 2001): 45–70, doi:10.1080/20014091091733.

CHAPTER 5

Effects of chewing on appetite, food intake and gut hormones: A systematic review and meta-analysis - PubMed (nih.gov)

Chewing and Attention: A Positive Effect on Sustained Attention (nih.gov)

https://pubmed.ncbi.nlm.nih.gov/24854804/

https://pubmed.ncbi.nlm.nih.gov/24854804/

CHAPTER 8

https://www.health.harvard.edu/staying-healthy/healthy-eating-plate

https://www.cnbc.com/2021/03/01/harvard-study-mix-of-fruits-and-veggies-linked-to-longevity.html

CHAPTER 9

https://fitfoodiefinds.com/healthy-pancakes-1-base-batter-6-ways/

https://www.delish.com/cooking/recipe-ideas/recipes/a51807/low-carb-breakfast-burritos-recipe/

https://www.wellplated.com/kale-feta-egg-toast/#_a5y_p=3422321

https://simply-delicious-food.com/easy-healthy-salad-sandwich/

https://www.bbcgoodfood.com/recipes/spiced-lentil-butternut-squash-soup

https://www.bonappetit.com/recipe/bright-and-spicy-shrimp-noodle-salad

https://www.bonappetit.com/recipe/lemony-salmon-and-spiced-chickpeas

https://www.lecremedelacrumb.com/one-pan-spanish-chicken-rice/

https://www.acouplecooks.com/shrimp-and-broccoli/

https://www.jamieoliver.com/recipes/chicken-recipes/grilled-chicken-with-charred-pineapple-salad/

https://www.delish.com/cooking/recipe-ideas/recipes/a36265/steak-dijon-recipe-ghk0214/

https://glutenfreeonashoestring.com/homemade-protein-bars/

https://www.modernhoney.com/6-healthy-superfood-smoothies/

https://drivemehungry.com/sweet-and-tangy-sticky-soy-glaze/

Printed in Great Britain
by Amazon